Indian Medical Science Series No. 160

AYURVEDIC MINERALS, GEMS AND ANIMAL PRODUCTS for Longevity and Rejuvenation

Dr. H.S. Puri, Ph.D.

Sri Satguru Publications
A Division of :
INDIAN BOOKS CENTRE
DELHI • INDIA

Published by
Sri Satguru Publications,
Indological and Oriental Publishers
A Division of
Indian Books Centre
40/5, Shakti Nagar,
Delhi-110007
India

Email: ibcindia@vsı l.com
Website: http://www.indianbookscentre.com

First Edition : Delhi2007
Second Edition; Delhi, 2007

ISBN 81-7030-850-X

DISCLAIMER: The information given in this book is for educational purposes only, and not for the treatment, mitigation, diagnosis of any disease or condition. The aut or/publisher are not responsible for use of various recipes, without the supervision of an Ayurvedic physician

Printed at Chawla Offset Printers, Delhi 110 052

CONTENTS

FOREWORD

सिद्धे रसे करिष्यामि निर्दारिद्र्यगदं जगत् ।

Nagarjuna, the father of *Rasashastra* asserted that he would make the word free from the poverty and diseases. He mastered the art of converting low metals into precious metals like gold and number of mercurial therapeutic preparations for eliminating diseases.

In brief *Rasashastra* means Ayurvedic metalo-mineral pharmaceuticals and therapeutics as such, it deals mainly with the drugs of mineral origin, their varieties, characteristics, processing techniques, properties and therapeutic uses. The term *Rasasastra* is composed of two words i.e. *Rasa* and *Sastra*. In general the word *Rasa* represents for many things, however in this context it has been used for two meanings. The first meaning is an "absorbable form of drugs" and the second meaning is "mercury". The word *Sastra* means the science or the "knowledge". Thus the technical term *Rasayana* means the science or the knowledge, which may teach to convert the drugs, irrespective of their nature (i.e. herbal, mineral or animal) in *Rasa* or absorbable form. As per the second meaning the term *Rasasastra* is to denote a science or the knowledge related to mercurial processing.

In the context of *Rasasastra* two term denoting concepts are generally referred to i.e. *Lohavedha/Rasavedha/Dhatuvedah* or *Rasayanavedah*. Actually these are the two main objectives of *Rasasastra*. A *Dhatuvedah* is converting low metals into precious heavy metals. **B** *Dehavedha* is making the body very strong, free from diseases, and stable for longer duration with the use of mercurial preparations.

The actual development of *Rasasastra* as an independent branch of learning and therapy was started from the 8th century A.D. But before that period in *Caraka* and *Susruta Samhitas* also there is a good deal of description of *prathiva* type of drugs, their processing techniques and their principles.

There is a need of standardization of preparation of metalo-mineral drugs (SOP) and also their validation for safety as there is an undue fear about the toxicity of these drugs. This therapeutic branch is neglected though it has high potentials.

Number of mineral, animal and marine products find place in ancient as well as in contemporary literatures of Ayurveda for therapeutic purposes. I am very happy that the matter is compiled and systematically presented in this book, "Ayurvedic Minerals, Gems and Animal Products for Longevity and Rejuvenation". I hope this compilation will be very useful for the students, researchers, academicians and doctors.

Dr. G. S. Lavekar
Director
Central Council for Research in Ayurveda and Siddha
Ministry of Health & Family Welfare, Govt. of India

PREFACE

Recent researches have indicated now that most of the items used for rejuvenation and longevity (*Rasayana*) may have antioxidant, immunomodulater, or adaptogenic properties, and by virtue of these effects, they help in stress, ageing and even in sexual inadequacies. *Rasayana* is a Sanskrit word, consisting of two parts: *Rasa* which means-extract and *ayana* is path. The primordial tissues of the body, formed by the assimilation of dietary items is called *Rasadhatu (rasa* is extract and *dhatu* tissue so *Rasadhatu* means the tissue formed by the extract of nutrients). The products, which improve the quality of this *Rasadhatu* by utilizing the extracts of the nutrients in a proper way are *Rasayana.* According to *Carak Samhita* (written about 100 AD), by the use of *Rasayana* " One obtains longevity, regains youth, gets a sharp memory, intelligence, freedom from diseases, lustrous complexion and strength (sexual) of a horse." This diverse action of *Rasayana* may be due to their property of modulating an endogenous system of the body, setting into motion a cascade of events leading to the multiple effects due to psycho-neuro-immunology. Some recent studies have shown that *Rasayana* act primarily on the components of the immune system such as macrophages and activate the cytokine network. Pretreatment with *Rasayana* is effective in protecting animals to a varying degree from different infections. If used after infection, with or without antibiotics, they reduced mortality as compared to the control. These have significant immunomodulater, cytoprotective and anticanerous effect also. Oral administration of four *Rasayana* preparations significantly increased total leukocyte count, bone marrow cellularity, natural killer cell activity and antibody dependent cellular toxicity in mice exposed to gamma radiation. These also reduced radiation induced lipid peroxidation in the liver. This action could be due to increased stem cell proliferation and effect on free radical induced injury produced by radiation. One of these *Brahma Rasayana* inhibited methyl cholanthrene induced sarcoma development in mice. They delay ageing, and strengthen the tissue to withstand both endogenous and exogenous stress by blunting stress induced rise in plasma steroids and suppression of peritoneal macrophage functions. In the case of obstructive jaundice it was seen that some of the *Rasayana* not only activate the immune cells of the liver but also increase bile flow into gut. The immune cells of the liver deactivate the endotoxins while bile salts in the gut adsorb the toxins. This reduced the movement of the toxin into circulation and prevented the complications associated with obstructive jaundice. When *Chavanprasha avleh*- a well known *Rasayana* preparation, was used in old age patients, there were immense beneficial effects.

Rasayana are of many types, and may consist of single herb (*ekdravy*) or may be compound preparations. The compound preparations may be prepared from a large number of herbs, minerals, gems and animal products. In my earlier book, a detailed account of herbs used as *Rasayana*, is given. In the present work other materials used as *Rasayana* are described.

In last a few decades, quite a number of books have been published on Indian medicinal plants, showing the importance of herbs in day to day life of various cultures, but very little information is available on the use of gems, minerals from various sources and also on the animal products. It is interesting to find that the use of the fresh flesh and organs of various animals is given in the Ayurvedic literature for various treatments and great importance is attached to them even now as a rich source of energy for the body but in *Rasayana* preparations these have been used to a limited extent. In various *Rasayana* preparations mostly animal products used are coral, shells, pearl, horns etc., which are rich in minerals, and musk, amber, civet, the fragrance of which has a strong effect on nervous system. The milk products and honey act as direct nutrients.

For minerals deficiency, many metals have been mentioned, but for the present purposes details of those items, which have *Rasayana* like effects, are given. In due course of time, some important gems also became a part of this treatment. All these water insoluble materials were processed in various ways to form complex organo-metallic compounds so as to make them bio-available. The processed minerals mainly consisted of heavy metals, which are now known to cause widespread damage to the immunity system, but all the minerals were used after processing and that also in compound preparations in a very limited quantity, which chelated these out of the body without causing any toxicity.

A general account of processing of these animal, mineral and gem has been given in the general introduction in each case.

Shilajit, which has recently come into prominence again, is a complex organo-mineral compound of unknown origin. With the further development of metallurgy and gemology, Ayurvedic physicians incorporated a number of these and other products in their compound herbal preparations. The result of all these activities is that now we have a large number of formulations used as *Rasayana*, both in the Ayurvedic classical literature and in the commercial products.

The therapeutic efficacy of most of the minerals, gems and animal products is not very well known at the present. It has been seen that these minerals and animal products, particularly mercury, fortify the therapeutic efficacy of the herbs but only further research will throw light on this not so well known aspect of ancient Indian medical science. It will give a new stimulus to search for new safe and effective therapeutic agents for some of the incurable diseases. Some of these non-herbal products are being used for last several centuries for wasting diseases and for rejuvenation (*kaya kalp*) purposes and there is every possibility that these may provide a new lead to the discovery of new therapeutic agents. Some recent surveys have indicated that information obtained from ethnopharmacological studies provide a better clues for search of new drugs, as compared to random studies of plants and chemicals

Dr. H.S Puri

MINERALS

INTRODUCTION

The science of metallurgy and geology was well developed in the pre-historic India. A frequent mention of metals is there in the ancient texts and historical records. The interesting thing is that most of the development on the medicinal uses of minerals was not developed in Ayurveda but in closed allied system *Siddha* which is mainly practiced in Tamilnadu and the adjoining areas in south India. The practitioners of this system of medicine are called *Sidhars*, and their achievement as *siddhi*. According to tradition, it was god Siva who gave knowledge of *Siddha* system to his consort Parvati, who handed it to Nandi deva and from there it went to *Sidhars*. Eighteen *Sidhars* seem to have existed in the long span of time. Some of them were well conversant with both Tamil (language of a part of south India) and Sanskrit. In the early stages *Siddha* originated and developed independently but later on, as happens with all types of knowledge, there was exchange between Ayurveda and *Siddha*, both systems sharing the knowledge of each other. Since *Siddha* system said to have originated by the knowledge imparted by Lord Siva, this system of medicine is sometimes known as *Siva sampradayam* (tradition of Siva) or *Sidha sampradayam*. On the other hand Brahma, who is the creator of universe, taught this science of Ayurveda to Prajapati to *Aswini devtas* so Ayurveda is sometimes called *Brahma* or *Arsha sampradayam*. From this it is evident that *Siddha* system was the creation of Dravids in south India whereas Aryans developed Ayurveda in the north.

In *vedic* era literature of Aryans, frequent references of processing of gold, silver, copper, tin, lead and non-metal antimony are found. In the *Siddha* system also since the earliest times mercury, sulphur, copper, arsenic and a variety of other minerals were used. The Ayurvedic author Carak and Sushrut (100BC to 100AD) were also well conversant with iron in the medicine. Carak even mentioned sulphur and arsenic and gave an account of their medicinal uses.

Kautilya (400AD) mentions that first iron and then gold metallurgy was developed. He gave an account of processing of these metals at that time. Nagarjuna, in medieval India, obtained the knowledge of use of minerals and the other toxic ingredients and inorganic substances of animal origin, used in *Siddha* and popularized their use in the northern India under the title "*Rasa sastra*". His teachings spread as far as Tibet, Mongolia and the other parts of Central Asia, where he is still probably known as Guru Padmasambhav. *Rasa sastra*, as we see now, is a specialized branch, which deals with animals, minerals, gems and toxic herbs. The aim of this *shastra* is to find out the compounds, which make the herbs act on the body in a faster and more effective way. *Rasa sastra* products are thus more powerful, as compared to pure herbs, even in low dozes, and are to be used under the supervision of an Ayurvedic *acharya* (medical specialist). *Rasa sastra* may be called "Indian Alchemy" in which mercury plays a dominant role.

In Ayurveda, both *dhatu* and *lauh* stand for metals. Now, the term *dhatu* in Ayurvedic physiology is mainly used for vital energy of the body (semen) and metals but the word *lauh* stands for iron metal only. For therapeutic use seven metals: gold, silver, copper, tin, lead, iron and zinc are mentioned. These are called *saptlouh* or *lauhsaptak*. *Dhatus* (metals) are a good conductor of heat and electricity and by virtue of these physical properties, they interact with the *dhatu* (vital energy) of the body to show their therapeutic effects.

As mentioned above, because of impact of *Rasa sastra* on Indian medicine, in ancient Indian metallurgy, stress was laid on the study of mercury because of its unique nature. It was not considered a metal but a divine blessing as it has power to react with most of the metals, minerals, gems and other substances. Because of this property, mercury was called a *ras* or a juicer or extractor or *ras raja* the king of extractors, as it could extract the therapeutic active constituents from an herb or mineral etc. by combining with it. The term *ras* became the center of all chemical activities and gave rise to a separate branch of ancient Indian medicine, *Ras tantra* (technology of mercury), which further developed into *Ras sastra* (science of mercury) and even *Rasayana,* which means the carrier of vital extracts from medicament or food etc. and *Ras shala* was the laboratory or the place of extraction (The term *Rasayana* is now is used for chemicals, and chemistry is called *Rasaynik shastra* or *Rasyanik vigyan*.)

Nagarjuna was the father of the science of mercurial chemistry and under his guidance this science developed so rapidly in medieval India that more than 300 ancient manuscripts on *Ras tantra* are available now. From 7th to 13th century knowledge about mercury was shrouded in mystery. Most of mercury technology was a guarded secret, monopolized by an extremist sect, known as *Tantaric*.

These perverted people developed their own moral philosophy and secret sexual rituals for a happy, long life and for attainment of salvation. Mercurials had a very important part in their rituals and red oxide of mercury (*sindur*) was a starting point.

Whereas alchemists in the other parts of the world at that time were concentrating on synthesis of gold, the Indian chemist devoted most of their energy to find out an elixir of immortality. The diverse antimicrobial property of mercury, particularly its ability to form complex compounds with sulphur, to kill most resistant types of microorganisms, which are causative factors of many chronic and obstinate diseases, and effect of mercury on the varied rejuvenating physiological properties of the human body, lead the ancient Indian physicians to believe that they have a tool of immortality in their hand in the form of mercurials.

These mercurials were often mixed with various herbs, animal products, minerals (both metallic and non-metallic) in various proportions, in different formulations for diverse physiological actions. Quite a number of ingredients were also used to suppress or modify the toxicity or side effects of mercury. The commonly used inorganic items, in addition to the metals mentioned above, were gems, animal skeletons or exoskeletons of the lower animals, sulphur, mica, alum, chalk, lime, saltpeter, potassium carbonate, sodium carbonate, borax, ammonium chloride, and various forms of common salt etc.

In addition to mercury Ayurvedic sages paid special attention to two more compounds *shilaji*t (complex organomineral compound of natural origin), and *banslochan* (silicic acid etc.). An account of *shilajit* is available in this book while *banslochan* has been described in book on *Rasayana* by Puri (2003)

PROCESSING OF MINERALS

The non-fleshy animal products like exoskeleton of marine animals, shells, bones etc, and various metals, gems and minerals are water insoluble, and hence cannot be assimilated by the human body. To make them water-soluble various recipes were developed by treating these with herbs, juices etc and then heating them so that they turn into partially water soluble, complex organic compounds.

It was customary to start the processing of medicinal raw materials after worshipping a particular deity, followed by washing of all the non-vegetable matters with water to remove the impurities sticking to them. The raw material was then treated variously with specific herbs or the other ingredients in various types of apparatus. In *Urdhavapatna yantra* (Fig.1A), the sublimed material got condensed inside the upper pitcher, whereas in *Baluka Yantra* (Fig 1B) the starting material was heated uniformly in sand in an airtight system. *Damru Yantra* (Fig.1C) is dumbbell shaped for uniform heating and mixing. In *Patal Yantra* (Fig.1D), for extraction of low melting point materials, the inverted bottle is heated at the top and sides, and molten liquid is allowed to drain in a fluid through the neck. In the *Dola Yantra* (Fig. 1E) the mineral is cooked into the decoctions of the herbs.

The various ingredients of a formulation were then subjected to the common method of beating and heating.

The raw material was usually enclosed in two crucibles, one above the other, sealed from all sides with clay and heated. Earlier the heating process was carried out in a pit, by burning cow dung cakes but now electric furnace is used. In some cases the process of heating and beating was repeated 100 times (*shatput*) but sometimes up to 1000 times (*sahastraput*). It was considered that minerals treated 1000 times have a better potency than those treated 100 times. The main precaution observed during this processing was that there should not be any particle of pure metal in the end product. The product so obtained is called "*bhasam*" which literally means ash, as the metals or minerals after this processing get converted into an ash like compound. In most of the translations of Sanskrit books into European languages, the word ash was frequently used for these processed minerals. Later it was observed that the minerals get oxidized by the above treatments, so these were referred to as 'metal oxides'. The recent chemical analysis have shown that the physico-chemical treatments of polyherbal, polymineral compounds result in the formation of quite a number of compounds and not oxides alone so in the present texts these organo-metallic compounds prepared from the minerals/metals are mentioned as "processed" instead of ash or metallic oxides.

In the case of poisonous plant materials and non metals, the word "*maran*" which means killing i.e. killing the toxicity, and "*shodhana*" meaning purification is commonly used in Ayurveda, which actually is a process of mitigation. In these cases, the toxic material is treated with boiling fluids and is not subjected to direct heat at high temperature.

GENERAL METHOD OF PREPARATION OF *BHASAM*

In the preparation of any *bhasam* (ash, processed products) of a mineral or any hard animal product, the first step is s*hodhna* (purification), and the second stage is *maran*- literal meaning killing (to deactivate the mineral by calcinations). By these treatments the metals lose their metallic texture and acquire an ash like appearance. In the case of diamond and mica, the product so obtained is called "*satva*". Generally the preparation of *bhasam* involves the following steps:

Bhavana

Any metal, herb or any other product when pounded with water, or a decoction or a juice to form a thick paste is called *bhavana*. Generally for *bhavana*, the herb and the mineral are taken in equal quantity. First one part of the herb is boiled in eight times of water till it is reduced to one eighth, after filtration, coarse powder of metal/mineral is added to this decoction.

Shodhna

The aim of this method is to remove the contaminants from the mineral so that the starting material is pure. For this either of the two approaches, given below are applied.

a) Samanya Shodhna

Common method is by heating and beating the metal or mineral into thin sheets, and immersing these sheets into a fluid medium like oil, juice, cow's urine etc.

b) Vishesha Shodhna

The starting material is purified by a special specific treatment in each case.

Marana

The method of deactivating the toxicity differs in each case depending on the nature of the starting material, but in general the purified material to be calcined is put into a stone mortar with the juices or extracts of the specified plants to form a uniform paste. From this paste, small flat balls of the mineral, depending on the nature of the material, are made and dried in the sun. These balls are then stored in a sealed clay tray. A pit is dug in the ground, and half of this pit is filled with cow dung cakes. The tray containing material to be processed in the form of balls is placed above these cow dung cakes in center of the pit and is covered over further with fuel cakes. The cakes are then ignited and allowed to burn, till they get extinguished of their own. When cold, the tray is taken out of ash, the contents of the tray are removed and made into a fine powder.

The heating operation in most of the cases now is carried out in the electric furnaces.

Characteristics of *bhasam*

According to the Pharmacopoeial Standards for Ayurvedic Formulations (1986) the *bhasam* as the finished product should have the following characteristics:

1. In the powder, there should not be any particle of a metallic luster.
2. When rubbed between index fingers, the powder should be so fine that it sticks inside the lines of the finger (as we see is the case of zinc salts).
3. It should be lighter than water. When sprinkled over cold water in a beaker, it should float.

4. When heated repeatedly, there should not be any physical change in final finished *bhasam* i.e. no loss of weight or change in colour etc. When heated in a crucible with equal quantities of honey and silver, *bhasam* should not react with silver to form a compound. It should remain separate.

FURTHER READING

The *Ayurvedic Formulary of India.* Ministry of Health and Family Welfare, Government of India, New Delhi.

Mahdihassan, S. (1992) *Indian Alchemy or Rasayana in the Light of Asceticism and Geriatrics.* Motilal Banarsidass, New Delhi (India).

Mukherji, B. (1998) *Wealth of Indian Alchemy and its Medicinal Uses.* 2nd Edition. South Asian Books, India.

Pharmacopoeial Standards for Ayurvedic Formulations. Central Council for Research in Ayurveda and Siddha, New Delhi (India).

M1 ARSENIC *(Sankhiya)*

Arsenic is one of the oldest poisons known to Ayurveda since ancient times. Earlier it was often used for homicidal purposes because of easy availability, desired effect in low dozes, not a distinct taste and easy incorporation in food materials. Tolerance to arsenic poisoning is well known and people have been known to develop a tolerance to it from a single large doze (acute poisoning) or repeated small dozes (chronic poisoning).

In Indian mythology, there is a frequent mention of young beautiful girls, fed with very small dozes of arsenic to start with and the dose was increased slowly so much so that by the time the girls reached puberty, they had accumulated large quantities of arsenic in their body and they would become toxic for others. These girls were known as "*Vish Kanya*", 'venomous girls' or 'serpent girls' and were used for enticing the victims for political reasons. Anybody coming in contact with them died of arsenic poisoning. It is also said that the persons who have excess of arsenic in their body if spit on a healthy person, he dies instantaneously.

Arsenic was also used as an intoxicant, and was said to make snake venom ineffective. It is probably mixed with opium to make it more effective. In medieval India some people developed the habit of addiction by snake- bite, arsenic in these cases acted as antidote to snake venom.

Medicinal virtues have also been ascribed to arsenic in various civilizations. Some springs containing arsenic in very low concentration in water are visited as a health resort even now. The water is said to have many curative properties including against some forms of cancer. The water is considered a blood purifier, and must be drunk freely along with the bath of the affected parts often by applying cloths wet with warm water from the spring.

In nature arsenic compounds are available in various forms. Common arsenic is As_2O_3, white arsenic (arsenious oxide) is As_4O_6 and arsenic penta oxide is As_2O_5 but in Ayurveda, arsenic trioxide (*sankhiya*) and compounds of arsenic and sulphur such as realgar (As_4S_4) and orpiment (As_2S_3) are commonly used. Realgar is orange scarlet in colour while orpiment is yellow.

The arsenic compounds in therapeutic dozes, act as a general tonic and alterative by increasing the appetite, and by stimulating the circulatory, respiratory and the nervous systems. These compounds help in certain kind of anemia, by increasing the number of red blood cells. They act as bronchial stimulants in bronchitis by increasing secretion and by dilation of capillaries. The arsenic compounds show their effect as an anabolic stimulant by combining with glutathione, an enzyme which retards oxidation and favours growth and weight. This fact was well known in the western world (Mansfield, 1937), and arsenic compounds were official in many pharmacopoeias of the world earlier. Before the discovery of the antibiotics, the arsenic salts also established their reputation as antimicrobial agents. They destroy *Spirocheta pallida*, the organism responsible for syphilis. Arsenic was also said to be effective against the malarial parasite.

USES IN AYURVEDA

As an antimicrobial agent

It has a strong antimicrobial and antiseptic effect. Earlier arsenic compounds were used before onset of malaria.

As an anabolic agent

It increases the metabolic rate of the body many times, leading to over consumption of food, digestion of fat and hard to digest food, and hence an increase in the weight, increase in the quantity of blood, heart rate, strength, respiration, and thus helps in chronic anemia, and sexual stress. It is prescribed with nutmeg powder in these cases. Arsenic plays an important role in metabolism of methionine- an amino acid involved in growth. The requirement is as low as 12 mcg, daily intake 140 mcg. The toxic level is 250 mcg/day.

In anemia

In the last century arsenic preparations were commonly incorporated in the formulations containing iron salts used for anemia.

As an antidote to poison

It probably acts as an antihemorrhagic agent against snake venom.

In chronic diarrhea

It helps when food passes out undigested.

In cancer

It has general type of anticancerous activity. In a type

of acute leukemia, the Chinese workers have shown that arsenic trioxide has a therapeutic effect.

As an immunostimulant

It is used for a variety of diseases commonly with *ghee.* Arsenic boiled in milk for a long time, till some of it dissolves, is prescribed in extremely low dozes in milk, as an immunostimulant in the beginning of rainy season, when the weather is quite mild or in low temperature conditions. Patient is given plenty of milk and *ghee.* For further safety use of *Triphala* is recommended.

If after the administration of arsenic compounds there is an urge to pass stools, gastric troubles or purgation then it is considered that the arsenic compounds are showing their effect.

AYURVEDIC COMPOUNDS

In Ayurveda, mainly the three forms of arsenic known as *sankhiya*, *hartal* and *manshil* are used.

Sankhiya

It may be white or red but usually white one is used, which is soapy to touch. It is a byproduct of metallurgical industry. Before use, it is processed by packing its coarse powder in a bag of thick cloth, and boiling this bag, for a whole day, in a mixture made from the milk of goat, *Amaranthus spinosus* juice or bitter gourd (*Momordica charantia*) juice or meat extract.

The compound so obtained, is said to be *tridoshnashak*, and is curative of all types of diseases due to *kapha.* If used for one month, it gives relief in respiratory diseases, and leprosy. It increases libido extensively. It helps in rheumatism, syphilis, fevers, anemia, controls tuberculosis in the early sages, is useful in angina and the other cardiac conditions.

In one of the preparations 125 mg *sankhiya*, and 15 gm black pepper is macerated in ginger juice for three days and pills of 125 mg are made. One pill twice daily is administered with ginger juice. As an anabolic agent, it is used with nutmeg

Hartal

It is sulphide of arsenic, and in nature is found in two physical forms

Flakes: which are golden in colour, lustrous, and soapy to touch

Solid: It is non-lustrous and considered, poor in quality.

Hartal can be manufactured artificially by heating 49 parts *sankhiya* with 24 parts of sulphur.

For medicinal purposes, 60 gm *hartal* is processed by macerating it with ten times its weight of latex of *Calotropis* spp., till a paste is formed. From this paste small cakes are made and dried in the sun. A crucible is filled half with bark powder of *Butea monosperma* and incinerated till ash is formed. Dry cakes of *hartal* are placed on this ash, covered with another crucible and heated for whole day till they turn off white in colour.

In another method, an earthen pot is compactly packed with the ashes of *Ficus* bark, *Cassia fistula* and *Euphorbea royleana*. The cake of *hartal* is placed on this ash and is covered over with more ash till the pot is full. The ash is compacted and an inverted clay pot is placed upon it. The sides are sealed with clay and the whole assembly is heated.

In the third method coarse powder of *hartal is* heated for four hours, one after the other in lime-juice, water boiled on smoked wood, and boiling water. The mineral so obtained is mixed with equal part of calcined mother of pearl, and macerated with aloe pulp till a paste is formed. It is made into small pills.

This processed compound is used in all types of sexually transmitted diseases, particularly syphilis, skin diseases, skin ulcer, acute and chronic skin eruptions, and many types of cancer. Doze: 30-60 mg

In a clinical trial, tablets of a preparation "*Bhootbhairav Ras*" which contained processed *hartal* (flakes) 48 mg, processed sulphur 19 mg, *Momordica charantia* 32 mg and *Tamarindus indica* 25 mg, when tried on the patients of epilepsy, along with adjuvant therapy, reduced the frequency and duration of the seizures (Paranjape, 1995).

Hartal not processed properly causes inflammation, pain, shivering, tingling sensation, poisoning of blood, and skin disfiguring which makes the whole body ugly

Mankiya ras

An important preparation of *hartal* is *Mankiya ras*, which is of two types.

i). First type of this product is made by macerating 100 gm each of purified *harta*l, *hingul* and sulphur in the juice of *Butea frondosa* flower, for one week. After drying, it is subjected to sublimation to obtain a red powder deposited along the sides of the upper container.

ii). A number of methods are used for the preparation of the second type of the product but essentially it consists of treating foil type *harta*l with the juice of wax gourd (*Benincasa hispida*) and sour yogurt. After washing and drying *harta*l is wrapped in mica sheets and heated for three hours till ruby red in colour. On cooling this gives rise to particles of *Mankiya ras.*

It is considered a good preventive agent for many diseases of old age, and a geriatric tonic for common diseases of skin and blood.

Manshil

It has a *hartal* like effects and can be manufactured by heating in a closed vessel a mixture of pulverized *sankhiya* 49 parts and sulphur 16 parts. The product so obtained is further purified by heating 8 parts of *manshil* with one part each of raw sugar (jaggery), ginger, processed iron and *ghee*

Doze of pure arsenic is 1-4 mg and for arsenic compounds 30-60 mg (lethal doze is 60 mg for arsenic and for arsenic compounds 125 mg and above)

ARSENIC POISONING

Despite the reputation of arsenic as a poison, it has actually very low toxicity in combination with some other metals. The average intake of arsenic is estimated at 1 mg per day mainly from foods but this is not toxic, this organic arsenic bound in foods or in Ayurvedic products is well tolerated by the human- body. On the average, there is about 10-20 mg of arsenic in human body. There is limited evidence for the carcinogenicity of arsenic in experimental animals. With chronic exposures, arsenic has an effect on chromosomes and carcinogenicity. Some bad effects have been observed with calcium arsenate, arsenites, or trivalent form of arsenic, used in industry but not with arsenic compounds used in Ayurveda. Arsenic may be essential and functional in humans in a moderate doze but higher levels may be toxic. It has been shown to be essential in rats in small amounts, which can tolerate much higher amount as compared to man. It is eliminated by kidney. Arsenic can accumulate when kidney function is decreased but most of it is excreted through feces and urine.

Possible effects of arsenic toxicity include hair loss, dermatitis, diarrhea, and other gastrointestinal disturbances.

SYMPTOMS OF ACUTE ARSENIC POISONING

According to Mansfield (1937) lethal doze of arsenic causes pain in abdomen, dryness of throat and difficulty in swallowing, abdominal cramps, vomiting with bile or blood, diarrhea with bloody stools, scant urine with blood, pulse rapid, weak and irregular, respiration slow, skin cold, cyanosis, collapse, spasms and convulsion, general muscular paralysis and asphyxia

In chronic arsenic poisoning the symptoms are: eye lids red and swollen, discharge from nose, skin eruption, pigmentation and exfoliation of skin, nausea and vomiting, abdominal cramps, hands and feet swollen, and muscles become paralyzed

TREATMENT OF ARSENIC TOXICITY:

In Ayurveda, *Benincasa hispida* (wax gourd) juice 250 ml with sugar candy and cumin seed 10 gm, three times a day is prescribed. Milk with honey quenches thrust and gives relief in nausea and inflammation

Lime water, if administered immediately after the poisoning neutralizes the effects of arsenic. According to Mansfield (1937) an arsenic antidote is prepared by adding a solution of ferrous sulphate to magnesium dioxide. The stomach of the victim should be washed, give emetics followed by mucilage of acacia or olive oil. Caffeine citrate or strychnine sulfate are given hypodermically.

Arsenic is excreted through feces, urine, saliva and tears. It remains in the body up to three weeks after the treatment.

CONTRAINDICATION

While using arsenic medications do not take salt, and hot and bitter items. Avoid all types of heat from fire or sun, and remain in a cool place.

REFERENCES

Mansfield, W. (1937) *Materia Medica, Toxicology and Pharmacognosy*. CV Mosby Co, St Louis

Paranjpe, P. (1995) "Bhootbharav Ras" in the management of epilapsy, *Deerghayu International* **11**:10-12.

M2 GOLD (*Suvarn, Sona*)

Gold is known since middle ages for health restorative properties. Even wearing of gold ornaments and touch of gold to human body in any way, as a ring, bracelet, necklace, a rub on the bald- head and milk in a golden pot or water with a gold piece in it, was said to give relief in certain ailments. Gold earrings were supposed to improve eyesight, and gold chain healed mumps. The alchemist in Egypt developed an elixir made of liquid gold, which had the ability to restore youth and perfect health. This knowledge spread all over the world and gold was said to have a direct effect on the heart, helping to improve blood circulation, rejuvenating sluggish organs especially the digestive system and the brain in the cases of nervous incordination. It was used to stimulate the nerves and stabilize body's temperature. It helped in cases of chills, hot flashes, and night sweats.

In western world, gold was used to bring good fortune, ward off evil spirits and to heal the sick. Historically gold had reputation as a "nervine"- a therapy for nervous disorder. During the 19th century, it was used for depression, epilepsy, migraine, impotence and menopause. It was observed that gold has milder side effects than mercury. In occasional cases treatment with gold produced an increase in vitality and intellectual faculties and had stimulating effect on the glands and sexual functioning. Gold was found to be an excitant, and a valuable remedy for melancholia. It induced in the patients a sense of well being. The patients felt more active and erotic. Gold fortified with silver and copper exerted a powerful influence on the nervous system. Nobel Prize winner bacteriologist, Robert Koch observed that the compounds made with gold, inhibited the growth of *bacillius* that causes tuberculosis.

Gold was valued in Asian medical systems also. A Tibetan medicine *Thanga baspam,* which has gold as an ingredient, is used as an aphrodisiac. In *Unani Tibb* (Greeco-Persian system of medicine) a gold- containing preparation, *Jawahar Mohra* is considered good for longevity. A processed gold preparation, *Poorna Chandrothyam*, is well known in *Siddha* System (a south India system of medicine), where it is used as a general tonic in anemia, tuberculosis, debility, epilepsy, neurasthenia, in drug addiction and for longevity. The ancient Chinese physicians were first to prepare and use red colloidal gold for longevity (Mahdihassan, 1985).

According to Ayurveda, gold imparts strength, longevity, attractiveness, and beauty to women. It is good for eye and heart, and provides desired nutrition to the whole body. It is a brain tonic, cardio tonic, a *Rasayana,* and antidote to all toxins of the body. It keeps away the stress developed by worry, anger, fear, sadness, unstable mind, depression, illusion, self-pity, inferiority, unconsciousness, and weakness. It calms the agitated nerves. It increases blood supply to brain, and thus helps in mental retardation and forgetfulness. It helps in symptoms like those of AIDS (Acquired Immune Deficiency Syndrome) and the other sexually transmitted diseases, in wasting disease, decay of bones, and inflammation of testes. In the last stages of a patient, when there is a question of life and death, gold with

Emblica fruit and *Acacia* bark is prescribed. Gold is also used for conception and as a *Rasayana* for 1-10 years old children. It increases the "*ojas dhatu*" (immunity). For a healthy life a golden rod dipped in honey is applied on the tongue of infants.

Ayurvedic physician earlier used gold in chronic infections as it has a very strong antimicrobial effect. During its administration the body temperature increases, probably due to a strong metabolic activity induced by it. If this temperature becomes unbearable the dose of gold containing product is reduced or stopped altogether. According to Ayurvedic physicians, gold has a cooling effect on the body and whatever heat is generated in the body, is due to destructive activity of gold on the microbes.

Gold can be used as such, or as follows:

a) **In the form of fine particles**: These are obtained by rubbing gold on rough stone. The powder obtained this way is antitoxic. It is good for eyes, and helps in impregnation.

b) **Gold foil (leaf):** These are prepared by hammering 22-23 carat gold ingots till a few micron thick. These are used for coating the pills or other surfaces. This may be used with sugar candy. These prolong life of human beings, impart vigour, and heal wounds.

c) **Gold chloride**: It is made by dissolving gold into acids. It helps in menstruation irregularity, diabetes, chronic bronchitis, dysmenorrhea, impotency, lunacy, hysteria, melancholia and schizophrenia. Doze is 2-6 mg.

For its administration, 125 mg of gold chloride is dissolved in 30 ml of distilled water. A doze of 10-12 drops is given in chronic cases. It should be administered with cooling drinks, syrups, and fruit juices. It is not to be used with any mercury compound.

d) **Shell gold** is prepared by macerating in a mortar, equal quantities of honey, salt along with gold foils. This mixture is transferred to a glass container and warm water is added to it repeatedly, shaken slightly, till all honey and salt are removed from the mixture, as seen by the taste of water. The mixture is allowed to remain in the glass container for sometime, till the golden particle settle down. The water above gold is decanted off with a dropper without disturbing gold at the bottom. The gold- particles are dried by heating slightly and dry gum acacia powder is added to it. Whenever required, it is mixed with water and used. It forms a fine coating on the surface.

Impurities of copper and zinc are often present in the gold, so in Ayurveda for medicinal purposes it is purified before use.

PURIFICATION OF GOLD

Cut gold foil into small pieces in a crucible, and add to it a mixture of hydrochloric acid, and nitric acid, in the ratio of 4:1, heat the crucible till all the gold foils get dissolved in the acids. Heat the solution further followed by treatment with oxalic acid solution. Pure gold in the form of yellow particles settles down. The pure gold so obtained is processed further.

Gold is also purified by heating small pieces of thin plates, immersing them in the lemon juice, heating them again and treating them further with fermented grains, followed by mixtures of rock salt and oil, cow's urine and yogurt milk, cow's milk and *triphala* decoction. The process of heating and cooling is repeated in each mixture

6-7 times. The gold so obtained is considered as purified gold.

SUVARN BHASAM

Many methods are used for processing gold into non-metallic product called "*bhasam*". The easiest way for its manufacture is to triturate equal quantities of purified gold and purified mercury with lemon juice and wash the contents with water. After this add marble powder, which should be half the weight of gold, and triturate the mixture further with lemon juice for three days, till a dry powder is obtained. Mix to this powder equal weight of purified sulphur and heat the mixture in crucible till no shining metallic particles are visible. Add to this mixture decoction of *Bauhinia variegata* bark and heat the mixture again. Repeat this process of addition of *Bauhina* decoction and heating three times. When this process is complete, gold *bhasam* in the form of violet colour powder is obtained.

Another simpler method is to take one part of gold foil, two parts of mercury, three parts of sulphur, and add enough lemon juice to moisten the whole mass. Heat this mixture in a closed crucible, and allow it to cool. Repeat this process 14 times. Gold turns into a dark brown powder by the treatment.

In another method, take 24 gm of gold foil purified as above. In a container triturate 6 gm purified mercury, 6 gm purified sulphur with the latex of *Argemone mexicana* and cover the whole mass with the golden foils to form a ball. In another container prepare a paste of *Bauhinia purpurea* bark and immerse the golden ball in it and heat the ball in a crucible. Repeat the process of cooling and heating seven times. By this treatment gold turns into an ash- like compound.

Amritkaran (nectarization)

The above processed gold is further purified by wetting and drying it six times each in *Abrus precatorius* juice, lime-juice (*Citrus lemon*), aloe pulp, and *Eclipta alba* juice. After each treatment gold is heated, cooled and is then subjected to next juice. In the end the moisture free product, so obtained, is stored in a cool place.

AYURVEDIC PREPARATIONS

Gold is an ingredient of classical preparations like *Braham Rasayana, Jawahar Mohra, Makardhawaj, Navratnakalp Amrit, Ramchuramani Ras, Suvaran Malini Vasant, Suvaran Vasant Malti, Vasant Kusmakar Ras, Vrahida Vangashwar Ras* (Puri, 2003). The other important products are:

Mrig-nabhi-yadi Vati

Take musk 2 gm, saffron 4 gm, cardamom seed 5 gm., nutmeg 6 gm, *banslochan* (bamboo manna, silica) 7 gm, mace 8 gm, gold foil 8 gm, silver foil 3 gm, and pearl paste 4 gm. Except musk, silver, gold foil and pearl paste, make fine powder of rest of the ingredients. Macerate all the ingredients in juice of *Piper betle* for 36 hours, and make pills of 125 mg each.

Doze: One or two pills with sweet cold milk.

Use: This compound can be used by healthy persons of both the sexes, as given below, as well as a geriatric tonic. It helps the patients of mental and nervous breakdown. It increases physical strength and mental power. It acts both on the nervous and arterial system but it is more effective in the case of men, as compared to women. It has a cooling effect so can be used even in summer both by men and women.

Use by men: Because of its cooling effect, it can be used by the persons of hot temperament in whom diseases have arisen due to 'heat' in the body. It helps the persons who eat hot spicy food, and overindulge in sex. It is very useful in sexually transmitted diseases, general lethargy, involuntary ejaculation, premature ejaculation and deficiency of semen. If impotence is due to blockage of flow of blood to penis and the adjoining area, it acts as a vasodilator.

Use by women: It provides strength to the brain, nervous system, sexual system and, makes body strong. During pregnancy or lactation, these beneficial effects are passed on to the child It pacifies all the symptoms of menopause

Kam Churamani Ras

Ingredients: *Mukta pishti* (pearl paste), *Suvarnmakshik bhasam* (processed iron pyrite), *Suvaran bhasam* (processed gold), *Bheemsani kapoor* (borneol), *Javitri* (mace), *Jaiphal* (nutmeg), *Vang bhasam* (processed tin) and *Rajat bhasam* (processed silver) each 25 gm, and fine powder of equal quantities of cinnamon (*dal chini*), and cinnamon leaves (*tejpat*) 110 gm.

Method: Mix all the ingredients in *Asparagus racemosus* (*shatawar*) juice, triturate for seven days and make pills of 60 mg.

Doze: 0ne to two pills, twice daily with milk sweetened with refined candy sugar (*mishri*)

Use: *Kam Churamani Ras* is a supreme aphrodisiac and a boon for urinary and genital diseases of both males and females. It is a good spermatogenic agent and shows good effect even at the age of 80 years. With its use even an old person behaves and acts like young man sexually. It helps in diabetes, urinary diseases, inflammation and acts as an antidote to blood toxicity. For women it is useful in menopause.

THERAPEUTIC USES IN AYURVEDA

The usual dose of the processed gold is 15-30 mg. (in Western medicine, the doze of pure gold was 1.95 mg to 5.85 mg, while the present anti-arthritic drugs the doze is 6 mg). Gold processed in Ayurvedic way is used as follows:

In the wasting diseases due to weakness

Gold *bhasam* with *Centella asiatica* juice, *Calamus* powder, *Asparagus* juice, and *Nardostachys jatmansi* decoction gives good results

In premature ageing

Suvarn bhasam with *Chavanparash, Makardhawaj* or processed mica is given.

As a mental tonic

Take gold *bhasam* with *Calamus*, *Tinospora,* ginger and *Asparagus* for six months

For strength and beauty

Take gold *bhasam* along with *Desmodium gangeticum*, *Pueraria tuberosa*, *Withania somnifera*, *Mucuna pruriens*, for three months.

For conception

Mesua ferrea with gold *bhasam* during menstruation induces and increases conception power in females.

As a spermatogenic agent

Processed gold (30 mg) when used for three months, with equal quantities of *Desmodium gangeticum* leaves, *Pueraria*, *Withania*, *Mucuna,* produces enough sperm to impregnate, even in a weak persons.

For ischaemic heart disease

An Ayurvedic compound preparation is used.

In cancer

Processed gold gives some relief.

PHARMACOLOGY AND THERAPEUTIC

Gold therapy is known as Aurotherapy and when used for arthritis, it is called Chrysotherapy. Potter (1894) mentioned that small doses of gold promote appetite and digestion, stimulate the cerebral function, produce a marked mental exhilaration, aphrodisiac effect in both sexes and a sense of well- being. The 1899 Merck's Manual list gold under aphrodisiacs. Hare (1912) observed that gold with common salt (sodium chloride) was a powerful sexual stimulant for erection. A mixture of gold chloride with sodium chloride was found to be an effective treatment for cocaine, morphine and opium addiction. Fomon (1920) found that gold preparations stimulate the nervous system and the sexual glands and were useful in alcoholism and opiumism. For alcoholism gold chloride with strychnine was used.

Use of gold in dentistry also became popular in that era and continues even now. American dentist use 13 tons of gold very year. It is non-toxic, non-corrosive metal, and can be shaped easily. It never wears, corrodes or tarnishes.

Recently gold preparations are recognized replacement for steroids in treating skin diseases (Thomas, 1987), asthma and in several forms of cancer (Fricker, 1996). It may affect the IgE immune response in asthmatic patients, which inhibits the release of histamine.

In an experiment, a gold compound blocked virus replication in infected cells. Gold instruments are applied to clear coronary arteries. Gold leaf is used in treating chronic ulcers as well as in surgery to patch damaged blood vessels, nerves, bones and membranes.

Compounds of gold were first used in the treatment of rheumatoid arthritis experimentally in 1927 and now are the basis of an accepted form of therapy. The gold compounds used in the treatment of rheumatoid arthritis in the modern medicine are: Auranofin, Aurothioglucose and Gold sodium Thiomalate. These compounds do not help in all the cases but most of the arthritic patient, get relief in joint pain, stiffness, swellings, bone damage, joint deformity and disability. Bajaj and Vohra (1998) studied the analgesic activity of gold preparations. Two Ayurvedic products were compared with anti-arthritic drug Auranofin in rats. Both products exhibited analgesic activity, which may be due to opiodergic mechanism of the preparations.

A commercial preparation (SUHART) consisting of oils of nutmeg and clove, black pepper, *Commiphora wightti*, rose and *Pandanus odoratissimus* extract, saffron, and processed gold and mica, reduced significantly requirement of an antiaginal drug. Twelve out of 13 patients of ischaemic heart disease showed significantly low angina frequency (Mitra, 1991).

Anticancerous properties of *Suvarn Ras Sindur* (gold processed in mercury) have been tested by Patil *et al.*

(1996). This product inhibited benzidine- induced degranulation of rough endoplasmic reticulum of liver and kidney of albino rats. It protected the induced toxicity by inhibiting lipid peroxidation and formaldehyde formation.

Earlier it was thought that gold compounds are not absorbed through oral route and require intramuscular administration at weekly interval but recent studies have shown that it causes stimulation of cortisol secretion, when used in a ring it passes through the skin and local lymphatics to nearby joints in sufficient quantity to delay articular erosion. Natural occurring gold is found in nervous and glandular tissues and behaves in some cases as a natural essential trace element and may change in concentration and correlation with certain diseases. It is found concentrated in glandular and reproductive tissue and in females its concentration cycles with the reproductive cycle. It is much higher in concentration in placenta than other tissues. It is richest in semen also (Richards *et al.* 2002).

TOXIC EFFECTS

Gold is toxic to living system. It gets accumulated in the body and is slowly excreted by kidney.

The toxic effects of gold include nausea, vomiting, glandular irritation, violent gastroenteritis, mental disturbance, convulsion, priapism, trembling and paralysis.

Gold preparations cause sores, pimples, blotches, tumours and ulcers but the sores readily heal up without any treatment

According to Ayurveda, if during treatment with gold preparations, symptoms of gold poisoning appear, then after vomiting and purgatives, give processed mica as an antidote followed by administration of honey or *Emblica*, till the toxic symptom subsidize.

Gold induced neuropathy (abnormal condition of peripheral nerves) is reported and in these cases, the patient recovered after cessation of gold therapy (Misra *et al.* 1987). According to Richards *et al* (2002) three forms of gold-induced neurological side effects have been recognized:

1) Painful neuropathy- insomnia and anxiety

2) Peripheral motor neuropathy

3) Encephalopathy- depression, delirium.

REFERENCE

Bajaj, S. and Vohora, S.B. (1998) Analgesic activities of gold preparations used in Ayurveda and Unani-Tibb. *Indian Journal of Medical Research*, **108**: 104-111.

Fomon, S. (1920) *Medicine and Allied Sciences*, Vol III. Appleton & Co NY

Fricker, S. P. (1996) Medical use of gold compounds, past, present and future. *Gold Bulletin*, **31**: 103-104.

Hare, H. A. (1912) *A textbook of Practical Therapeutics*. 14th edition. Lea & Febiger, Philadelphia.

Mahdihassan, S. (1985) Cinnabar-gold as the best alchemical drug of longevity, called Makradhawaja in India. *American Journal of Chinese Medicine.* **13**: 93-108

Mahdihassan, S (1992) *Indian Alchemy or Rasayana. In the light of Asceticism and Geriatrics*. Motilal Banarsi Das, Delhi (India).

Merck's 1899 Mannual of the Materia Medica, NY. Merck & Co (reprint 1999)

Misra, R., Mahesh Chandra, Karm A.M. (1987) Acute polyneuroptahy complicating Ayurvedic drug therapy containing gold- a report. *Indian Medical gazette*, **121**: 281-282

Mitra, D.K. (1991) Suhart vs placebo in ischaemic heart disease. *Medicine and Surgery*, **30**: 33-34.

Mukherji, B. (1998) *Wealth of Indian Alchemy and its Medicinal Uses.* 2 volumes. South Asian Books, India

Patil, S., Kanasde, A., Kulkarni, P.H. (1996) Evaluation of anticarcinogenic potential of Kachnar Guggal and Suvarn Ras Sindur in albino rats. *Deerghayu International*, **12**:7-11

Potter, S.O.L. (1894) *A compend of material medica, therapeutics and prescription writing with especial reference to the physiological action of the drugs.* Sixth edition 1902, Blakiston & Sons, Philadelphia.

Puri, H. S. (2003) *Rasayana: Ayurvedic Herbs for Longevity and Rejuvenation*. Taylor & Francis, New York and London

Richards, D.G., McMillin, D.L., Mein, E.A. Nelson, C.D. (2002) Gold and its relationship to neurological/ glandular condition. *International Journal of Neuroscience*, **112**: 31-53

Shastrina, K N (1979) *Rastringani* (in Hindi) Motilal Banarsi Das, Delhi.

Thomas, I. (1987) Gold therapy and its indication in dermatology. *Journal of the American Academy of Dentistry.* **16:** 845-854.

M3 IRON PYRITE *(Suvarnmakshik)*

It is iron bisulphide, and was sometimes substituted for gold in Ayurveda, because of its brass-yellow appearance. Before use, the mineral is purified by boiling it in lemon juice with one third of its weight of rock salt in an iron vessel till red hot. On cooling it is macerated with oil or goat's urine and incinerated till ash like. It is used as an anti-inflammatory and antihepatotoxic agent, particularly in the liver damage caused by quinine.

It is also used as *Satva,* made by heating equal quantities of *Suvarnmakshik* and sulphur in a shallow iron pan for twelve hours. On cooling, half the quantity of sulphur added earlier along with similar amount of borax are put in to this mixture and whole mass is heated in a crucible till a copper like red product is obtained. From this *Satva*, another product *Suvarnmakshik Satva bhasam* is prepared by macerating with lemon juice 60 gm each of *Suvarnmakshik Satva*, mercury and sulphur for the whole day. This mixture is dried in sun and then incinerated at a high temperature in a crucible.

It is considered a good *Rasayana* and panacea for incurable disease, and as an invigourating tonic for longevity.

M 4 MERCURY (*Parad, Para*)

The discovery and use of mercury started from *Siddha* system of medicine in south India. In this system mercury is considered the physical embodiment of the invisible internal fire (*tejas*). According to *Siddha*, mercury provides incredible amount of *tejas* to an organ and increases the metabolism several times.

In Indian mythology, origin of mercury is linked with Indian god Siva. It is said that while having sex with Parvati, just at the verge of ejaculation, Siva was disturbed by demons, so he ran after them, while doing so he ejaculated his semen on the earth, which gave rise to mercury, while the menstruating blood of Parvati is the source of sulphur. Siva explained to Parvati virtues of his ejaculate: mercury, who in turn spread this information all over the world.

In Indian alchemy mercury symbolizes the union of *Siva* and *Sakthi* (Parvati), and it is termed as *Siva beej* (the seed of Shiv) and sulphur *Parvati beeja* (the seed of Parvati). It signifies the universal law of creation, that is, unless both female and male gametes do not unite there will not be any further creation. The practitioners of *Siddha* system of medicine (*sidhars*) considered that the same phenomenon is applicable for the creation of a new effective medicaments also i.e. union of components of opposite nature. Because of its source of origin, mercury is hot, strong, volatile, dynamic while sulphur has opposite characteristics. It is cold, weak, frigid and static. Both mercury and sulphur neutralize the bad effect of each other and in Ayurvedic formulations both are mostly used together

The ancient practitioners of *Siddha* system, recognized five forms of mercury, which have now been identified as: 1) the pure metal as such, 2) red sulphide of mercury, 3) red oxide of mercury, 4) mercuric chloride (mercury per chloride) and 5) mercury sub chloride (calomel). It was said that used in any form mercury is life force or essence of life.

Nagarjun in the 3rd century or so conducted further research on this element, and developed many compounds of mercury mainly combining sulphur and mica with it. Because of its assumed divine origin and peculiar properties, mercury became a cult object of a mysterious religious sect *Tantra*, in which the priest class, the *Tantarics,* exploited it further and used it, particularly the red oxide of mercury (*sindur*), which signifies the menstrual blood, in various rituals. In *Rasa sastra*-the art of *Tantaric* alchemy, mercury is equated with semen and is considered as a living substance or a living being.

Mercury in Sanskrit is called '*parad*' or in short' *para*' - an agent, which keeps all the diseases away. The other Sanskrit synonyms also characterize the properties of this metal. It is called '*rasa*' which means juicer or extractor, which by it catalytic action extracts maximum therapeutic compounds from other medicaments and thus increasing their bioefficacy. In this way it may act as a panacea for many incurable diseases. Because of this supreme property it is also referred as *rasraj* or the king or the best of all for making various compounds, readily available to the body for cure. It is very reactive so is called *chapal.* The other names for mercury mean 'an element of great strength', and 'capable of digesting every thing in the body'. It was said that mercury changes the human appearance in old age the way it changes the metallic characteristics of gold and silver.

In Ayurveda it has been strictly laid down that only very pure form of mercury should be used in medicine. Lead is its common admixture in the nature but sometimes a small quantity of lead is added intentionally in mercury to prevent its loss during storage

PURIFICATION OF RAW MERCURY

Technology for processing mercury was highly developed in medieval India, and several methods involving all kinds of herbs and techniques were employed for its purification. Out of these a simple method for purification of starting material is as follows.

Macerate mercury with lime (calcium) for three days, and after that pass it through a coarse cloth. To the filtered mercury add equal weight of garlic, and half the quantity of common salt, and macerate the mixture till garlic paste turns black. Wash the whole mass with home made dilute vinegar. The mercury so obtained is said to be free from most of the extraneous materials, and is processed further, as given below, for use as a medicine.

It has been emphasized in Ayurveda that mercury not processed in a proper Ayurvedic way has no therapeutic efficacy and is toxic. In Ayurveda eighteen steps have been recommended for the proper purification of mercury for use in *Rasayana* and *Vajikarna* preparations, but usually the following eight steps are followed.

Savedna (subjecting to vapours)

Make a paste of mixture of long pepper, black pepper, *Plumbago zeylanica*, dry and fresh ginger, salt and *triphala*, home made mild vinegar and store the paste in *Dolayantra* (Fig. 1E). The weight of the paste of herbs should be l6th times of the weight of mercury to be treated. Mercury is tied in a cotton cloth and is hanged in the pot in such a way that it gets immersed in the above paste and vapours from the paste react to it from all the directions. The whole system is heated for the whole day. For next two days mercury is further processed by repeatedly washing it with the same type of paste, draining the earlier one and adding the new one. It is said that this treatment removes most of the impurities from mercury.

Mardan (trituration)

It is a process where the mercury obtained from above is macerated with salt, pure carbon (obtained from the smoke of the house), *Brassica juncea*, turmeric, garlic, ginger and *triphala.* These should be 1/l6th part of the mercury.

Murchan (to make unconscious).

Mercury in the third step is made inert by macerating it seven times, first with aloe, then with *triphala,* and last of all by *Plumbago zeylanica* root. By these treatments mercury gets rid of all the ill effects (*doshas*), and becomes inert.

Uthapan (regeneration)

Pure mercury from the above mass is regenerated by treating it with an acidic medium such as juices of citrus fruits, and home made dilute vinegar solution, for twelve hours, followed by washing with pure water.

Trividhpatan (sublimation)

In the fifth step, mercury is mixed with ferrous sulphate solution, washed with water and subjected to sublimation. By this treatment metallic contaminants like tin and lead remain behind in the pan while the pure mercury evaporates and gets deposited in the inner side of an inverted pot.

Bodhan (revival)

By sublimation, mercury becomes inert, so to reactivate it, it is packed in cotton cloth and dipped in boiling saline water at low heat.

Niyaman (to bring to the order)

The mercury obtained after *bodhan* is boiled in the decoction of garlic, *Eclipta*, tamarind, *Cyperus scariosus*, and ammonium chloride.

Sandipan (to reactivate)

In *Dolayantra* (Fig. 1E), mercury is boiled with the dilute solution of vinegar for six hours, which makes mercury reactive enough to form therapeutically active compounds.

COMPOUND PREPARATIONS

It is said that when combined with sulphur, mercury loses its side effects. If mercury, purified as above, is treated by weight with equal part of sulphur, then it is effective against ordinary diseases only, if with two parts of sulphur then for chronic diseases, with three parts of sulphur it imparts vitality to the body, with four parts of sulphur it gives energy to the body, increases memory, power, and strength, with five parts of sulphur it cures all the diseases and worries, and with six parts of sulphur it becomes a panacea.

It has been observed that the use of mercurial compounds with sulphur even for long time has no deleterious effect on the body, but those without sulphur lead to mercurial poisoning.

For preparing the above compounds of mercury with sulphur, all of the sulphur is not mixed in mercury in one step but in six divided doses. To a required quantity of mercury in a cup of clay or iron in *Balukayantra* (Fig. 1B), first part of sulphur is added to mercury and the mixture is heated. When sulphur starts melting, another part of purified sulphur is added and heating is continued, till fourth and fifth parts get molten. In the end sixth part is mixed till the whole mass is homogenous. The compound is cooled afterwards.

AYURVEDIC PREPARATIONS

When mercury is mixed and triturated with sulphur, a black sulphide is formed, but if a mixture of mercury and sulphur is heated, then red sulphide is produced, which vaporizes and condenses at the top of the vessel. This condensate on grinding turns red but by repeated pulverizing, the fine particles so formed impart a peculiar luster to it.

The various forms of mercury, as mentioned earlier are used extensively in Ayurveda. Some of the mercurial preparations are recognized in Ayurvedic Pharmacopoeia, while others are used by individuals and the pharmacies at their own level.

AYURVEDIC PHARMACOPOEIAL PREPARATIONS

Parpati or *Parpatika*

For the preparation, equal quantity of purified mercury and sulphur are molten in a pan and pressed between banana leaves. This preparation, when used increases the metabolic rate in the body.

Kajjali

When the purified mercury is triturated with half, equal, one, two or three parts of sulphur in pestle and mortar, a lustrous black product is obtained which is called *kajjali.* The finished product is tested for free particle of mercury, by suspending the paste in water and by allowing it to dry. If there is any free mercury, visible as shining particles, the mixture is processed again.

It is said that *Kajjali* pacifies all the three *doshas* of the body, and helps in the induction of sexual power. It boosts the activity of herbal formulations, so is sometimes added for their fortification as in the case of *Sooksham triphala*, where *Kajjali* is said to enhance the effect of *triphala.*

Parad Bhasam

It is prepared variously by triturating equal part of mercury and sulphur in the presence of herbal materials and then heating it, till a black mass is formed without any particles of free mercury in it.

One of the simplest methods of preparation of this product is to macerate mercury, sulphur and latex of *Ficus benghalensis* in a strong pot of clay. The whole mixture is heated slowly for the day and stirred constantly with twig of *F. benghalensis*. On cooling, next day a lustrous black product is obtained.

Use: It is said to keep the digestive system in order. It increases strength, vitality, sexual power and libido. It is a supreme geriatric tonic, and is a boon for amorous men. It fortifies the therapeutic efficacy of the other products.

Yellow *Bhasam*

Another form of the *bhasam* is prepared by macerating equal parts of mercury and sulphur in the juices of the herbs, and then the whole mixture is incinerated till a yellow product is obtained.

Raskapur (mercuric chloride)

Macerate together, in a pestle mortar 60 gm each of purified mercury, common salt, and ferrous sulphate. Fill this mixture in a glass funnel and place it in the *Balukayantra* (Fig. 1B) and heat for six hours. *Raskapur* will get deposited along the sides of funnel by sublimation. Citric acid or lemon juice is added to the end product as a preservative.

It is an effective antimicrobial agent, and is a strong diuretic. It removes excess of water from the body, and toxins from the liver. Even very dilute solution of this compound has an antiseptic property so was widely prescribed earlier for the sexually transmitted diseases, where it was administered both externally and internally.

Ras Sindur (red sulphide of mercury)

For the manufacture of this compound many methods are employed but all essentially consist of macerating sulphur and mercury in the ratio of 1:6 in some medium like aloe juice. When dry the whole mass is filled in a hard glass bottle and heated in *Dolayantra* for seven days, till red sulphide of mercury is formed.

It is considered a supreme aphrodisiac, and panacea for all diseases. It is said to keep the whole nervous system in order (antidepressant effect). It cleans body by regular bowel and urinary excretion. It is also used for fortification of the therapeutic activity of various herbal combinations.

As an aphrodisiac, pulverize ten gram each of *Ras Sindur*, *Withania, Anacyclus*, nutmeg, mace, camphor, *Calamus*, and *Cannabis* leaves. Mix equal quantity of sugar to this fine powder, moisten with water and make pills of 500 mg each. On drying cover the pills with silver foil.

Use one pill with the juice of fresh radish root.

Doze of *Ras Sindur*: infants 5 mg, toddler 20 mg, child up to six years 40 mg, up to 12 years 60 mg, and adult 125 mg.

In a study, rats under normal conditions and those subjected to cold stress of 4 hours everyday for a week, were administered *Ras sindur*, and their metabolic parameters such as blood urea nitrogen, creatinine, lactic acid, blood sugar and cholesterol were studied. It was seen that there was a significant increase in all the compounds except cholesterol, where there was a decrease. These changes were more marked in stress group. Estimation of sugar revealed initial hypoglycaemic effect in both groups. In a study when *Ras sind*ur was administered 40 mg/kg for 6-12 weeks to rats, it made their body more sensitive to changed conditions. Its effects were opposite to that of herbal adaptogens (Srivastava *et al.*, personal communication).

Makardhawaj

It is another form of *Rasa Sindur,* but during the manufacture of this product gold is used as a catalyst. A further modified form of *Makardhawaj* is called *Sidh Makardhwaj.*

Ingredients: Mercury 4 parts, sulphur 16 parts and gold 1 part.

Method of Preparation: Triturate gold and mercury in a pestle and mortar made of stone, followed by sulphur, till a grit free, lighter than water, lusterless, black mass called, "*kajjali*" is formed. Sometimes juice of red cotton flower and aloe pulp is added during triturating. The paste so formed is filled in thick glass bottle, sealed and heated. In the beginning the lid of bottle is kept open for the escape of sulphur vapours, but after sometime, the mouth of the bottle is closed, and bottle is heated further. By the action of the heat on the mixture, a red coloured powder is formed which gets deposited along the inner sides of the bottle, while gold remains behind at the base of the bottle. For the collection of both red coloured powder (*Makardhawaj*) and gold, the bottle is broken.

In about 1930 a German company E. Merck, introduced in India, red sulphide of mercury, manufactured by their own method and sold it under the name *Makardhawaj*, but Ayurvedic physicians at that time did not find this preparation as effective as the one manufactured by their traditional method by incorporating gold

Chemical analysis of *Makardhawaj* revealed 13% sulphur and 80.2% mercury in it, but there were no traces of gold in the final product.

Another preparation *Sidh Makardhawaj*, which is said

to be stronger than *Makardhawaj* in action, is prepared by taking gold 1 part, mercury 2 parts and sulphur 4 parts.

Makardhawaj is sometimes used as an ingredient of many polyherbal, polymineral compound preparations. One of these, a compound aphrodisiac product, is prepared by taking one part each of camphor, nutmeg, black pepper, clove, *Makardhawaj* and one tenth part musk. The pills of 10 grain (65 mg) each are made from this mass.

Dose: One pill wrapped in betel leaf with milk

During the use of *Makardhawaj,* use as much milk and fat as can be digested. As it is hot in effect, it is better to use this preparation in winter.

Hingul (Singraf)

This is prepared by macerating in a rotating drum, eight parts of sulphur and 42 parts of mercury to get a lustrous powder. This powder is fed to a crucible having another tight fitting crucible on it. The sides of these crucibles are sealed with clay. On heating this pair of crucible, soft *Hingul* gets deposited under the side of the covering crucible, from where it is collected. The pair of crucibles is heated again and again till all the *Hingul* is obtained. The product so obtained is first macerated with ginger or lemon juice seven times and after that is washed in water to get a red, soft, lustrous powder

Use: It is said to suppress the diseases due to *pitta.* It is a strong anabolic, detoxifying agent and induces *agni* in the body. It increases strength, intelligence, clears skin making it lustrous so is used in leprosy. It helps in all types of diseases due to *ama* and *vata.*

Note: For all mercurial preparations the maximum dose is 120 mg.

TABLE 1

A comparative study of the composition of different mercury and sulphur containing Ayurvedic preparations

	Rasa Sindur	Kajjali	Bhasam	Makra dhawaj	Sidh Makar dhwaj	Hingul
Sulphur	6	1,2,3	1	16	4	8
Mercury	1	1	1	4	2	42
Gold	-	-	-	1	1	-

AYURVEDIC FORMULATIONS

In addition to the above, mercury in various forms, is an ingredient of quite a number of Ayurvedic products such as *Madanodya Modak*, *Vish Rasayana*, *Amrit Rasayana, Luxmi Villas Ras*, *Vrhadavangeshawar Ras*, an account of which is given earlier in the book (Puri, 2003). Here some other formulations are given, which are as follows:

Sidhard Amrita

Lord Shiva is said to have developed this product. In this product 50 gm of *Hingul*, wrapped in thick cotton threads on all sides, is immersed in a pot containing 200 ml onion juice and 50 gm *Ficus* latex and is heated till all the water evaporates and *Hingul* forms a solid mass. On cooling, this mass is taken out, placed in other pot and covered- over with 25 gm clove powder. This clove covered *Hingul* pot is placed in a small pyramid like structure formed by 300 gm of *Semecarpus anacardium* fruit. For making this pyramid *S. anacardium* fruits are arranged in such a that conical part of the fruit is towards inside and broad side towards outside. The adjoining area around the fruits is plugged with clove powder, and the whole assembly is incinerated till burnt completely. On cooling, to the solid mass of *Hingul* is added ten times its weight of *ghee*, and it is incinerated again. When cool, *Hingul* is made into a fine powder with pestle and mortar.

Use: A 65 mg doze of this product is prescribed in paralysis, acute hepatotoxicity, in persistent impotency and is considered a panacea for other incurable diseases.

Gunjajiwan Ras

Make a coarse powder of *Abrus precatorius* seed (the seed is in two forms, one is bicolour black and red, and the other is off white in colour, out of these white variety is more toxic so bicoloured variety is preferred for medicinal purposes). Store the powder in a cloth bag and boil it in milk for three hours. Dry this powder and macerate 20 gm of it, along with 20 gm of *Rasa Sindur* and 40 gm of marijuana (Cannbi s) with water to form a paste. Make pills of 250 mg each.

Use: It is a good anabolic agent and increases libido enormously.

Triloksamohan Ras

Take 150 gm *Cannabis* leaves, and 12.5 gm each of processed *Hingul*, red sulphide of mercury, processed black mica and camphor, and 25 gm each of *Tribulus terrestris*, *Mucuna pruriens*, *Pistacia* galls. Macerate this mixture, seven times with *Cannabis* juice, followed by juice of rose petals till a thick paste to form pills of 375 mg each is obtained.

Use: It increases memory and has immense sexual

power, it creates maximum libido, desire, and prolongs the time of ejaculation.

Pushapdhanav Ras

Take equal quantities of processed mercury, lead, iron, mica and tin, and macerate them with the juices of *Datura*, *Cannabis*, liquorice, and *Salmalia* bark, to form a thick paste for making pills of 250 mg each.

Prescribe it twice daily with milk, *ghee*, butter or honey.

Use: It is a good tonic for urinogenital system. It increases libido, power, and mental alertness. It helps in insomnia, sexually transmitted diseases, and in impotence due to diabetes.

MERCURIAL POISONING

Mercury readily diffuses in the body and is a protoplasmic poison even at very high dilution. It increases the number of red blood corpuscles and lessens their coagubility. It alters the shape and function of proteins, hormones, antibodies, haemoglobin and enzymes. It suppresses immune system and body's defence against infection and disease. It appears that toxicity and side effects of mercury compounds are very much like tropane alkaloids (*Datura* spp.), and the side effects of both can be treated in the similar way.

According to Ayurveda, if during the administration of mercurials, excessive heat is generated in the body then cold water is sprinkled on the head followed by application of a paste of *Santalum album* wood. The patient should be kept in cool air, in a pleasing, cooling and soothing environment during the day, and under the open sky during night. If burning sensation in the chest region persists, then patient should be immersed in a tub full of cold water, and should be kept there till all symptoms subsidize. If the patient feels mental weakness then Ayurvedic preparations *Drakshaasav, Ashwagandharishta* along with the other nutrients, having a cooling effect on the body are given. In the case of acute dryness of mouth (thirst) coconut water, yogurt, milk or other thirst quencher are prescribed. Certain vegetable and cereals should be given as food. No vegetable oil is allowed but product from cow's milk can be taken. The vegetables which have diuretic action and which may drain mercury from the body are avoided.

The poisoning symptoms of excess of mercury in the body are: burning sensation in the mouth and stomach, pain in abdomen, vomiting, diarrhoea, salvation, hemorrhage from the lung, albuminaria, hematuria, retention of urine, delirium, and apoplexy.

If any of the above symptoms is observed during the use of mercury products, take the following steps:

1. Give an emetic immediately, followed by administration of a large quantity of milk.

2. Give powder of *Emblica officinalis* or bark of *Acacia nilotica* with hot water. It is very effective

3. Give purified sulphur with milk. If available, juice of *Piper betle* leaves may be added to the milk for additional benefit (mercury immediately reacts with protein in milk rather than that in the mouth).

4. In traditional treatment of mercury poisoning, a fluid prepared by 800 ml of juice of each of *Piper betle* leaves, *Eclipta, Ocimum* and goat's milk, is rubbed over all parts of the body for two days followed by a cold bath.

M5 MICA (*Abhrak*)

In nature, mica occurs in the form of white to grayish white lustrous foils or thick sheets. In Ayurveda, four varieties of mica: white, red, black and yellow are recognized but mainly transparent (white) mica is used. The yellow variety is very heat resistant and is considered a good geriatric tonic. This mineral is insoluble in water and can bear a very high temperature, so to make it bioavailable for the human systems, it is processed in various ways to form *bhasam*.

PREPARATION OF *BHASAM*

Mica is purified first by boiling in *Triphala* (A mixture of fruits of *Emblica officinalis, Terminalia chebula* and *T. bellerica)* water and after that it is soaked in lime juice and heated till all the flakes of mica get separated. These flakes are then triturated with *Amaranthus polygamous* juice to form a thick paste, which is then allowed to dry for a week. The mica flakes by this treatment become brittle and are crushed with hand and are sieved through a cheese-cloth (muslin). The powder at this stage is hard, heavy, very fine and black in colour. This powder is further treated with cow's urine and heated in a crucible and pulverized. This process may be repeated hundred times or sometimes even a thousand times to obtain the *bhasam*. It is said that by this repetitive process of heating and beating the potency of the *bhasam* increases many folds. A *bhasam* prepared by 1000 times of treatment is considered superior to that prepared by 100 times.

In some cases for the preparation of *bhasam* the mica is treated one after the other by *Calotropis* latex, *Ficus* latex, *Euphorbia* latex, *Solanum nigrum*, *Tribulus terrestris*, *Achyranthes aspera*, *Ficus benghalensis* buds, *Ocimum*, banana stolon and cow's urine by first making a tablet from the mixture of mica and a herb, and after that heating and grinding it. After 100 such treatments, mica powder turns into a reddish colour powder. The best product is red, fine to touch and without any shining particles.

A compound is prepared by mixing fine powders of this processed mica with *Trikatu* (long pepper, black pepper and ginger), *Embelia ribes, Emblica officinalis*, juice of *Cannabis indica* and pills of 250 mg each are made.

THERAPEUTIC USES

It is considered as an alterative and hematinic. It helps in respiratory diseases like chronic asthma and tuberculosis. It gives strength in old age and during disability. It is used for rejuvenation, youthfulness, inflammation in intestine, in the last stages of tuberculosis, wasting diseases, bone porosity, chronic bronchitis, hepatotoxicity and for delaying death. *Abhrak bhasam* stimulates metabolic activity in tissue cells, and acts as an aphrodisiac and restorative. When used along with long pepper and honey, it shows better effects.

Mica with mercury is said to be more effective as compared to the product obtained above. Many methods are used for this purpose but the simplest is to take mica 4 parts, borax 1 part, macerate these in the juice of any of the root used under the name of *safed musli* (*Asparagus sarmentosus*, *Chlorophytum arundinaceum*) and heat, till a brown coloured product is obtained. This brown powder is triturated with equal parts of black sulphide of mercury, before use.

Mica treated with mercury, is considered very cooling in effect, sweet, oily, and good for hair growth. It vitiates *tridosha* and is a good *Rasayana.* It imparts immense sexual power, youthfulness to the whole body and systems. There is no product, which can compete with it as an antiimpotence agent and as a geriatric tonic.

The therapeutic effect of mica may be due to supply of silica to connective tissues

TOXICITY

Mica not processed properly causes inflammation, lung damage, and chronic skin diseases.

CHEMICAL STUDY

Mica is mainly silicate of aluminum but after the treatments as given above, it changes into reddish brown, smooth powder, which on analysis showed iron 20.3 to 20.90%, aluminum 12.03 to 12.55%, phosphate (as PO4) 1.64%, magnesium 7.90 % and silica 35%, besides other compounds.

M6 SILVER (*Rajat, Chandi*)

In Ayurveda silver in the form of very thin foils, as an organometallic compound *(bhasam)* and silver salt is used. Very thin foil of silver is very commonly used. It is said in India in one year about 13 British tons of silver is consumed for edible purposes. Silver foil is made by hammering silver ingots in the intestine of oxen and the other animals. For this purpose intestine of the animals is pulled out, and washed to remove blood and the other animal remains. A silver block is placed in the middle of these bound intestines, it is pounded with wooden sticks till so thin that it sticks to the rice paper. The very thin silver foil so obtained is called *vark* or *varkh* (in Urdu it means page). This foil is used for decoration of a large number of Ayurvedic pills, silver coating of tablets and for decoration of candy balls or even a common masticator, *pan*.

Silver salt, silver nitrate is made by the common method of treating silver with nitric acid, while for preparing *bhasam*, many methods are used. In a common method silver foil is treated with twice its weight of cinnabar and the mixture is subjected to sublimation, which separates mercury from the mixture, and a black coloured *bhasam* is left behind. It consists of about 84% silver and 16% sulphur. In another method, fine powder of silver foil is heated with an equal amount of purified mercury, sulphur and aloe pulp, till the whole mass turns into ash. When heated further, it turns red. After cooling it is dipped in lime- juice.

USES IN AYURVEDA

Silver and silver containing compounds are considered *Rasayana* in Ayurveda. Earlier in the royal families it was customary to use silverwares for household purposes, and even poor people wear silver ornaments now.

For medicinal purposes silver foils or silver nitrate can be used as such or these are processed further by heating them on charcoal till red in colour. These are then immersed in lime- juice one by one with a pair of tongs. By this treatment these product turn soft. Silver foils may also be processed with arsenic salts. In one of the methods equal quantity of silver foils, made into small pieces, along with pure *hartal* and sulphur, are heated in a crucible till a black lustrous compound is obtained. It is said that during this process arsenic part of *hartal*, acts as a catalyst only, and escapes in the air.

Silver is considered a supreme *Rasayana,* useful for *vata pitta prokopa.* It is cooling in effect and helps in the diseases caused by hotness and *pitta* in the body. It is said to be a cerebral tonic and is of immense use to the brain-workers. It gives nutrition to the brain and increases memory. It calms the agitation of mind, helps in depression, cowardice, memory problems and mental illnesses. It helps in wasting diseases due to sexually transmitted diseases (syphilis and gonorrhoea), diabetes and various types of inflammations, and also in gangrene when the skin turns black. It has a good effect on impotence caused by sexually transmitted diseases and by constriction of the veins and arteries of the genital area. It imparts a fine texture to the skin and provides energy to all parts of the body.

Dose: 30-120 mg as per age, condition, strength of the patient and weather.

THERAPEUTIC USES

Silver in low concentration (colloidal silver, where particle size is .0003 to 0.5 microns, is said to be more effective) is a powerful wide spectrum antibiotic. It destabilizes the enzymes used by the microorganisms for respiration, so cripples virus, fungus, bacterium and other unicellular pathogens. In 50-200 parts per million levels, over wide range of pH, silver salts are able to do the job. Trace amounts of silver are prophylactic in action as they strengthen the immune system. It rapidly subdues the inflammation and promotes healing. The major uses of silver are:

As a general tonic

If processed silver is used with *Desmodium gangeticum*, *Mucuna pruriens*, and *Asparagus racemosus*, continuously for two months, it helps in all types of weakness in the body and makes the body strong

As a beauty aid

When used with *Emblica* fruit, processed *Semecarpus anacardium*, ginger and saffron, it makes women more beautiful.

As a cooling agent

In headache and cardiac problems, which are said to originate by excessive heat in the body, silver foil with *amalaki* (*Emblica officinalis*) fruit preserve is said to have a cooling effect on the body.

METABOLISM

Silver is excreted from the body in the form of silver sulphide through grayish black feces and through sweat but some of it gets deposited in kidney and liver.

TOXICOLOGY

According to a 1992 report by the Environmental Protection Agency (EPA) of the United States of America (USA), silver can be harmful to humans if eaten in a more than a miniscule amount (i.e. more than .005mg/kg per day). It is a bioaccumulative metal, once consumed silver lodges in the body fat and nervous system for life. Silver can cause lung and throat lesions and can spark infections and abdominal pain. It can also turn skin gray or black- a condition called argyreia, which has been observed in some people who consumed colloidal silver.

The result can be more disastrous if the so- called silver *vark*, adulterated with lead is used or they are made from lead or other metals like aluminum. Lead is known to cause brain damage to children

M7 SULPHUR (*Gandhak*)

Sulphur is known for a long time as an effective agent against skin diseases, but according to the Ayurvedic physicians it has a profound effect on the other systems of the body also. In alchemy sulphur is soul or individualized essence. In Indian mythology, sulphur is menstrual flow of Parvati. Mercury is semen of Shiva, and it is sulphur, which can control, Shiva's incredible potential.

Sulphur is available in various forms but in Ayurveda it is used after special process of purification. In this process a hard glass bottle is filled with sulphur, and a sieve is fixed in place of stopper at the mouth of this bottle. The bottle is inverted and is heated from above as in *Patal Yantra* (Fig. ID) so that the molten sulphur flows down in a container filled with milk, where it solidifies. This is purified, treated or processed sulphur. When this sulphur is washed a hundred times with water, it becomes odourless.

THERAPEUTIC USES

Treated sulphur is a digestant, laxative, tranquilizer, and *Rasayana*.. It cures leprosy, skin ailments, bronchial diseases and intestinal inflammation. It calms sudden bowl movement in the morning and excessive flow during gastroenteritis. If used for a long duration in prescribed dose, it improves eye- sight. It acts an antidote to poisons by metals like mercury and lead.

Usual dose of sulphur is 125 mg-1000 mg.

The various recipes and specific uses of sulphur are as follows:

As an anabolic agent

Take equal quantities of 10 ml of *Celastrus* oil, 10 gm *Calamus*, 10 gm fresh butter, and 30 gm powder of treated sulphur (deodorized by heating and cooling one hundred times). Use 250 mg of this product daily for one month. It makes a person strong, brave and disease free. It increases eyesight, contentment, and vital fluid.

For strength and vitality

a) Mix equal quantities of sulphur with young roots of *Salmalia malabarica*, take 250 mg of this mixture with milk sweetened with sugar, for one month.

b) Mix equal parts of treated sulphur, long pepper powder, and *Terminalia chebula* powder. Take one gram of this mixture with 4 gm *ghee,* and honey for three months. By its use body becomes strong and vigorous. It improves eyesight.

c) Mix equal amount of sulphur and *Emblica officinalis* powder. To this mixture, add juice of *E. officinalis* fruit and dry, add juice again and dry. Continue this process seven times, followed by similar treatment, seven times with *Salmalia malabarica* root juice. Take one gram of this preparation daily with sugar, milk and honey for 30 months. It imparts sexual vigour and increases libido in old men.

d) Mix fine powder of *Butea* seed in goat's milk and dry the mixture. Add to it one sixteenth part of treated sulphur and extract oil by heating the whole mass in *Patal*

Yantra (Fig. 1D). Smear 250 mg of this oil on *Piper betle* leaf, and sprinkle on this oil 125 mg of red mercury sulphide (*Rasa Sindur*). Rub both oil and mercurial vigorously on the leaves till the mixture turns black. Wrap the leaf and give to the patient for chewing. It is a supreme *Rasayana* It provides extreme sexual energy, strength to the body and cures bronchial diseases.

As a spermatogenic agent

a) Half gram treated sulphur when used with warm water for one month increases semen. After six months use it improves eyesight and changes texture of skin to golden yellow.

b) Make a homogenous mixture by taking one part of treated sulphur with nine parts of sugar. Take 125 mg of this mixture with pure water in seminal deficiency and for vitiation of semen (low viscosity, and putrid odour). By this treatment semen becomes viscous, and quantity of normal fertile sperms increases.

As a rejuvenator

a) Make a mixture of equal parts of fine powders of *Triphala (Emblica officinalis, Terminalia bellerica* and *T. chebula* fruits), *Ecliptaalba* and treated sulphur. Dose 2 gm per day for a month. It makes face wrinkles free and keeps hair black.

b) Macerate purified sulphur with *Eclipta* juice, let the mixture dry, moisten again with this juice three times, and use it with one gram of *T. chebula* powder with butter fat *(ghee*) and honey, in the morning for two months. Eat light food in limited quantity. This preparation defers old age and induces youthfulness.

c) Pulverize *Triphala*, *Eclipta* and sulphur to form a homogenous mixture. Two gram of this mixture when used for one month prevents premature graying of hairs and wrinkles.

AYURVEDIC PREPARATION

Gandhak Rasayana

Heat equal quantities of *ghee* and sulphur in an iron utensil till they form a uniform fluid. While hot, pass this molten mass through a cheese cloth (muslin) in a pot containing milk. On cooling, wash sulphur thoroughly with water and powder it. Add to this powder, decoction made from the mixture of cardamom, cinnamon, cinnamon leaves, *Mesua ferrea, Eclipta*, juice of *Tinospora*, and fresh ginger and dry the whole mass. Repeat this process of treating with decoction and drying eight times. The final product, so obtained is *Gandhak Rasayana.*

Dose: 1 gm with sugar.

Uses: It stabilizes *tridosha*. It imparts youthfulness and vigour. It is a good spermatogenic agent. It gives relief in swollen testes, and keeps all the skin diseases away. It helps in digestion, dysentery, gastroenteritis, diabetes, and all digestive problems. By using it for six months hair get darkened.

SIDE EFFECTS

Sulphur containing preparations appear quite safe. The excess of sulfur in the body, up to 80 per cent, gets excreted in feces, and the rest in the urine and sweat.

CONTRAINDICATIONS

While using sulphur- containing preparations, acidic, alkaline, and salt items, legumes, leafy vegetables, anger, worry and sex should be avoided.

M8 TIN (*Vang, Kalai*)

A few decades ago it was a common practice in India to get coatings of tin on the brassware used for cooking, as it is non-corrosive and resistant to natural acids. At that time it was available in the form of shinning, soft metallic coil. It was sometimes substituted by lead. In Ayurveda, tin is used in some important medicines after processing.

PROCESSING OF TIN

To the molten tin in a crucible is added one fourth of its weight of potassium carbonate and tamarind seed. The mixture is agitated continuously with an iron rod, till the whole mass is reduced to a powder.

In an alternative method limewater is added to molten tin from the top at a distance, through a small hole in the pot. Molten tin is always stirred with a spoon like structure having a long handle. The person operating the system must be far away from the crucible because if any fluid is added to the molten tin, then it shows vigorous boiling accompanied by liberation of splinters of tin, which penetrate deep in the body and may cause severe burns if proper precaution is not taken. Fumes of tin are also toxic.

With the above methods, tin turns into a powder. This powder is washed with cold water and treated with limewater or yogurt- milk or aloe juice and dried by heating. The process of addition of fluid is repeated seven times when lime-water is used and three times each when yogurt and aloe is used. It is essential that the end product is alkali free as tested with litmus paper. If not, then it is washed with fluids again. It is then pulverized to obtain a grayish white powder, mainly consisting of tin oxide.

For preparing *vang bhasam,* this prepared tin is molten in a slightly curved iron pot and one-fourth quantity of its weight of *Achyranthes aspera* or *Ficus* bark, dry powder is added to it slowly and whole mass is shaken with an iron spoon. The process is continued till tin loses its metallic luster. It is covered with a clay pot, and heated for the whole day. At the end of the operation, it appears as a dark red molten mass. On cooling this, an off white coloured powder is obtained.

USES IN AYURVEDA

Processed tin (*vang bhasam*) is considered an excellent preparation, which never fails to show its effect in diabetes, nocturnal emission and other types of sexual inadequacies. In Ayurveda it is said that it acts against urinogenital diseases the way lion acts against herd of elephants. It is also used in bronchial problems, in liver malfunctioning, as an anthelmentic, for increasing gastric secretions, and as a cure of tuberculosis. It is considered hot in effect slightly anti-*pitta*, as it aids digestion, and increases vital power. In sexually transmitted diseases, it cures skin diseases by detoxifying and purifying the blood.

In the case of women, it provides desired energy in the body which helps in menstruation problems, in back-ache due to scanty menstruation, in dysmenorrhoea, amen-orrhoea, and in sterility due to lack of ovulation.

In males it exerts its beneficial effect on neuromuscular system, the weakness of which causes impotence, seminal deficiencies, involuntary and nocturnal emission. It has a spermatogenetic effect. It provides desired energy for the whole process of sperm formation and thus helps in azoospermia, and oligospermia. It increases the quantity of spermatic fluid. If due to some reasons, body produces dead sperm leading to putrefied semen, then it revives the sperm production system.

According to an Ayurvedic concept, the men who consume sour, sweet, and hot fatty diet or indulge in excessive sex, suffer from premature and nocturnal emission because of the overheating of the nervous system, leading to hypersensitivity of sexual organs to various stimuli so much so that a minor sexual fancy may lead to ejaculation without providing pleasure. This conditions lead to stress and depression in man, who considers it as a loss of manhood.

Tin helps in the other urinary conditions like polyurea, which is said to be due to bad food habits. It provides desired energy to urinary, genital and connected nervous system, leading to regulated flow of both urine, semen or menstruation flow.

It appears that tin like mercury, acts in the same way on the body as tropane alkaloid found in many Solanaceous plants, as it dries all the secretions. It pacifies the oversensitive nervous system but keeps the brain active.

Some of the recipes containing the processed tin are as follows

In backache (of women)

Mix fine powders of *vang bhasam* 125 mg, nutmeg powder 500 mg, *ashwagandha* 500 mg, and give this mixture with honey.

In involuntary ejaculation

a) Take *vang bhasam* 125 mg, coral paste 125 mg, *Piper cubeba* powder 500 mg, mix all the items and take with honey

b) Take *vang bhasam* 125 mg, *shilajit,* 500 mg, mix both and use with cow's milk.

In seminal deficiencies

a) Take *vang bhasam* 500 mg, *Tinospora* starch 500 mg, *shilajit* 250 mg, mix with butter and sugar.

b) Take *vang bhasma* 125 mg, processed mica 125 mg, and *Bombax malabaricum* root 2 gm.

c) Take *vang bhasam* 125 mg, with 2 gm nutmeg and honey.

In impotence (If due to excessive, uncontrolled- ejaculation)

Take *vang bhasam* 250 mg, pearl paste 125 mg, *ashwagandha* 2 gm with cow's milk.

In leucorrhoea

Mix *vang bhasam* 250 mg and 125 mg ash of stag horns in pomegranate juice or sugar. With the use of this mixture the ovulation becomes normal.

As a geriatric tonic

Take *vang bhasam* 250 mg, processed lead 125 mg, processed mica 125 mg, with honey.

As an antidiabetic agent

Take *vang bhasam* 125 mg and *shilajit* 500 mg

As a brain tonic

Mix *vang bhasam* 125 mg, processed mica 125 mg and *brahmi* powder 2 gm

In skin diseases

Mix processed tin with sulphur and apply externally.

For delaying the time of ejaculation in premature ejaculation

Mix 125 mg *vang bhasam* and 5 gm *Cannabis* powder, in honey and use with cold milk.

(This preparation may be useful in hypersensitive skin, anxiety and tension)

AYURVEDIC PREPARATIONS

Vajikark (Aphrodisiac) I

Ingredients: Pulverize fifty grams each of ginger, long pepper, black pepper, *Terminlia chebula, T. bellerica, Emblica officinalis*, cinnamon, *Piper cubeba*, cinnamon leaves, sandal-wood, *Trapa bispinosa*, *Nigella sativa, Ptychotis ajowan* (Indian thyme) and twenty five gram each of mace, clove and processed tin. Mix thoroughly.

Use one teaspoon, with milk, twice daily.

Vajikark (Aphrodisiac) II

Pulverize 100 gm each of *Withania somnifera,* ginger, cinnamon leaves, cardamom, and *Terminalia chebula,* with ten gram processed tin and 5 gm saffron

Use half teaspoon with half- teaspoonful sugar candy and milk

Swapanmehantak vati

Ingredients: Pulverize tin 25 gm, soap nut (*arishtak*)

kernel 50 gm, and sugar 50 gm. Triturate all items with water, and make pills of 375 mg each

Dose 3-6 pills thrice daily with water.

Uses: In nocturnal emission, take two pills three times a day and skip meal in the evening. It is also used in the diseases of urinogenital system, diabetes, low viscosity of semen, azoospermia, nocturnal emission, and for delaying the time of ejaculation.

Suvarnvang (Golden tin).

It is sulphide of tin. It is manufactured by heating together, in a thick glass bottle, tin foils, mercury, acid, salt, sulphur and ammonium chloride. On cooling golden coloured particles are formed.

Dose 125-250 mg

Use: It is used in place of processed tin for strengthening the urino-genital system of both the males and females. It is a good rejuvenator, tonic, and induces health and vigour in the body.

In diabetes

In an experiment, when 20% suspension of this compound was given to normoglycaemic rats, significant hypoglycaemic effect was noticed.

In impotence, as a rejuvenator

It is prescribed with 4 gm powder of *Mimosa pudica* root or *Withania somnifera* leaf juice.

For boosting memory

It is given with the juice or decoction of *Centella asiatica*

In spermatorrhoea

It is used with *Piper cubeb* powder

TOXICOLOGICAL STUDIES

Tin is present in small amount in human organs and a normal adult man contains about 352 mg of it. Tin when ingested orally in low dozes is safe but the vapour of the metal, cause pneumonia like symptoms. It is poorly absorbed from the alimentary tract of man and is chiefly excreted with faeces with a slow elimination in the urine. Some part of it is retained in the liver, kidneys, bones and brain.

Long term use of tin has no side effects. High dozes for months cause paralysis. The LD *iv* is 100 mg tin, death occurring from CNS (central nervous system) and GI (gastro-intestinal) tract injury. Spleen and liver appear mostly affected. 75-500 ppm of tin in food products caused vomiting, diarrhoea, fatigue and headache. 200 mg/kg produced severe gastro-intestinal symptoms. Tin compounds are immunotoxin.

According to Ayurveda, tin if not processed in a proper way or made from impure metal, causes leprosy like disfiguring of the skin. Excess of it may lead to diabetes, inflammation, and diseases of the heart and of the blood.

REFERENCE

Joshi, Suresh, P., Gode, K.D., Chakravarthy, B.K. (1988) Effect of Swarn Vanga in madhumeha in albino rats. *Ancient Science of Life*, **8**: 30-37.

M9 ZINC (*Yashad, Justa)*

In ancient India, zinc was obtained by suspending fine powders of raw- minerals in an emulsion of water and oil. By this method all heavy materials settled down while the light impure zinc get separated in the oil. This crude metal was further purified by heating. Now for Ayurvedic medicines, pure metal obtained from mines is processed in Ayurvedic ways and used

PROCESSING OF ZINC

It is processed by first heating it to such an extent that it melts. After this lime water or latex of *Euphorbia* (dendroid forms) or milk are poured on this molten metal slowly. The process is repeated seven times and the end product so obtained is neutralized with weak acids.

It is also processed by treating it with sulphur and mercury. Sometimes arsenic (*hartal*) is also added to the mixture. In another method zinc is heated on an iron pan till it melts. This molten metal is treated with fresh *Azadirachta indica* leaf juice or powder, and stirred with *A. indica* twigs till the whole mass turns into a powder. The pan is covered with a lid, heated further for 4 to 5 hours and allowed to cool. The crust like zinc so obtained is immersed in water, crushed with hands, and filtered after 3-4 hours. The water insoluble part is boiled in the pulp of aloe, and made into small balls. These balls are subjected to a very high temperature followed by a low temperature, 10-11 times till a yellow coloured compound with a red hue is formed. This is pulverized to a very fine powder (200 mesh).

USES IN AYURVEDA

Zinc processed above is said to be bitter and cold in effect. It gives relief in diseases due to *kapha, pitta,* provides strength, intelligence, and helps in polyurea, respiratory diseases including bronchitis and tuberculosis and problems of digestive and urinary systems. It has an astringent effect and thus it heals wound, dries sputum and the other excretions from the body as in abscesses and profuse menstruation. It cures eyes diseases when applied externally.

Zinc may be used as zinc chloride and zinc sulphate by treating it with hydrochloric acid and sulphuric acid respectively. The compounds so obtained are much more astringent in action as compared to Ayurvedic processed zinc.

Processed zinc is used in the preparation of a *tridoshnashak* compound with small cardamom seed, cinnamon and *Cinamomum* spp. leaves.

In involuntary ejaculation, a mixture of 125 mg processed zinc and 125 mg *shilajit* is used. In acute diabetes the above mixture is mixed with the starch of *Tinospora cordifolia*. In tuberculosis, when the symptoms get aggravated, equal weight of pearl paste and *Adhatoda vasica* syrup is added to the mixture. When administered with *Ras Sindur*, it gives relief in mental fatigue and restlessness.

Doze: Processed zinc 65-125 mg with honey, butter or sugar. (The United States Recommended Dietary Allowance for zinc is 5 mg for children under one year old, 10 mg for age 1-10, 15 mg for adults, and 16-19 mg for lactating mothers.)

PHARMACOLOGY AND THERAPEUTICS

Zinc is present in every cell of the body. Excess of zinc during growth period increases growth hormone levels in the blood which enhances the growth rate, increases the number of cells in the body, promotes absorption of fat, and elevates insulin activity

Present studies have also shown that there are about 300 zinc dependent enzymes in the body and it is involved in the production of nucleic acids, DNA and RNA. Its deficiency in infants in pre adolescent stage leads to growth retardation, impaired learning and failure of sexual system. It not only has antioxidant property, but protects the immune system and is a major disease fighter. Zinc deficiency has been one of the factors in the atrophy of thymus gland in children and in old age. The gland produces less of hormone. This results in increased susceptibility to infection.

Zinc is required for testosterone production so it helps in infertility if due to low testosterone levels. Zinc supplements stimulate sexual maturation and improve fertility. The deficiency of this metal in male leads to impotence, decrease libido, along with the other side effects like uremia. Oysters have long been prized as a booster of sexual potency, this effect may be due to zinc. Prostate gland contains high concentration of zinc. Zinc deficiency has been linked to low sperm count and infertility in males and in females during pregnancy and may produce serious birth defects and foetal loss.

Zinc may be short in the body due to excessive alcohol consumption, cirrhosis of liver, diarrhoea, kidney disease, cystic fibrosis, rheumatoid arthritis and the other inflammatory conditions. Zinc helps in absorption of vitamins, sexual performance, fights stress, fatigue mental dullness, lowers cholesterol, blood sugar abnormality, growth retardation, delayed wound healing, immune response, hair loss, emotional disorders, and recurrent infections. It reduces the symptoms of the common cold, such as cough, sore throat, hoarseness of throat, nasal congestion, sneezing, and fever. It inhibits prostaglandin metabolites implicated in common cold and may induce the production of immunostimulant interferon. It has been a popular remedy for common cold, when used in a lozenge.

AYURVEDIC PREPARATION

Balark Gutika

This preparation is used for the care of infants and young children.

Ingredients: Pulverize equal quantities of processed zinc, processed coral, processed stag horn, processed *singraf* (a form of red sulphide of mercury), dehydrated borax, dehusked black pepper, saffron, and *Hedychium spicatum*. Moisten the powder so obtained with water and make pills of 65 mg each.

Method of administration: Make paste of one pill in mother's milk, or make a paste of fine powder of *Embelia ribes* seed and the above pill in milk, let the child lick it, followed by feeding by mother.

Use: This pill provides nutrition to all the systems of the body of infants and young children, makes their body strong and healthy, and keeps common ailments like mild fever, bronchial and digestive problems, and worms away.

It particularly helps in malodour, diarrhoea and scanty yellow coloured urine.

TOXICOLOGICAL STUDIES

Zinc if not processed properly in Ayurvedic way gives rise to symptoms seen in leprosy, tuberculosis and diabetes. Since it is excreted through feces and urine, it appears that digestive and urinary systems are most affected by its toxicity.

GEMS

INTRODUCTION

According to some Ayurvedic astrological theories, planets have a profound effect on human physiological systems/ body parts. Human destiny including health is controlled by planets. The planetary configuration, at a particular moment determines good or bad health of an individual. A particular planet may not be good for a particular organ of the human body at a specific time. We cannot have any control on planets, as they are far away from us, but we can pacify their ill effects or substantiate their good effect by the use of gems. Thus health/fortune, gems and planets are interconnected with each other. Each planet is associated with a gem and, it is considered that the use of that particular gem can pacify or suppress the bad effects of a corresponding planet, which in turn heals an organ/system of the human body. In all nine gems (*navratna*) are recognized, which consist of seven rare precious stones, pearl and red coral. In modern sense the word gem stands for minerals but ancient Indian considered both red coral and pearl, though animal in origin, as gem, because these are found at the sea bed, have mineral like appearance and are hard to find.

In due course of time, Ayurvedic concept of human health became dependent on astronomy and gemology (Table 2). It was considered that each gem radiates certain waves, which have a beneficial effect on the body as the gems have property to absorb rays of certain wave-length, while reflecting the others.

(Note: It has been observed that infrared ray emitting stones can be used, to treat cancer and degenerative diseases. These rays help in tumour inhibition by inactivating cancer cells while activating healthy cells at the same time. Among several studies, the stones of 4-14 micron wavelength demonstrated remarkable efficacy in treating various diseases).

On the basis of the above assumption, the gems are worshipped, or tied on a particular part of human body on some auspicious moment as per the planet configuration at that time, or are dipped in water according to a particular ritual and that water is drunk. The commonest practice is to use the gems in the ring. For this purpose, gems of a certain minimum weight, colour and good in clarity (flawless) are used and mounted on the ring of gold, silver, copper or even an alloy of eight metals (*asht-dhatu*). The mineral/gems used for such purpose are cut in such a way that their tapering lower side touches the skin of the finger.

Sometimes the gems are prescribed for internal consumption in the form of a paste (*pisht*i). Since these are water insoluble minerals, for better bioavailability, in some formulations, they are incorporated after heating them at a high temperature along with various herbs and minerals. The product so obtained is ash like in appearance and is called *bhasam*.

The main idea behind gem therapy appears to be to provide micronutrition of rare elements to the body as these gems are obtained from diverse sources; from deep sea to the high mountains, and sometimes consists of rare elements not normally found on the crust of the earth.

TABLE 2

Relationship Between Human Body, Planets and Nine Gems (navratna)

Part of human body	Planet	Gem
Flesh	Sun	Ruby
Hair	Moon	Pearl
Skin	Mars	Coral
Blood	Mercury	Emerald
Bone	Jupiter	Topaz (yellow sapphire)
Marrow	Venus	Diamond
Fat	Saturn	Blue Sapphire
Semen	Rahu (north node)	Amethyst or Hessonite, Garnet
Vitality	Ketu (south node)	Chrysoberyl, Cat's eye

GEM STONES IN THE WESTERN WORLD

As per western thoughts, gemstones are not connected with planets but crystals and gemstones have always been used by the healers because of their energy activation property. Gem- therapy is used for strengthening the body and resolving tissues and patterns. It is said that gem heal human beings by opening, running and programming human auras. Stones with clear colours have stronger healing energy, as do the stones with larger size. For their beneficial effects gems can be placed under a table, on the table, on the picture of gods or can be tied to the body during meditation. They can be used in ornaments or carried in the pocket during sleep or kept under the pillow.

They may be immersed in water or a fluid and water/fluid may be used as a drink . They may be smeared with honey and suck. The key to using stone is to place them into aura (body's energy field).

GEM STONES IN AYURVEDA

Traditionally in yoga, gemstones are used to activate *kundalini*, which is a hypothetical dormant, innate (implanted by nature) power of divinity within an individual, which lies at the base of the body.

In Ayurveda, a single gem may be used in medicine but commonly a mixture of nine stones called *Navratna* are incorporated as one entity in some Ayurvedic products. The important preparations containing these nine gems are *Jawhar Mohra, Navratan Ras*, and *Navratan Kalp Amrit*.

In addition to the common nine gems, sometimes some other semi-precious stones are also used. The detail of all theses important gems is as follows:

G1 CAT'S EYE or CHRYSO-BERYL (*Vidura, Lahsunia*)

It is a smooth stone and before use is boiled in the decoction of *triphala* three times and is processed as in the case of diamond or ruby.

Astrologically it is the gem of planet *Ketu* of Indian astrology. When its (*ketu*) effect is weak, it causes doubt, uncertainty, poor discrimination, poor concentration or lack of insight. It is the planet of ultimate spiritual awakening.

It is considered very cooling in effect. It pacifies *pitta* and increases digestive power, memory and strength. It is laxative and good for eyes. Dose 15-60 mg.

Note: In *Siddha* system of medicine, lapis lazuli is considered *vidura*.

G2 DIAMOND (*Heera*)

It is the purest form of carbon and the hardest substance known. Its hardness is 10 and specific gravity 3.5. It is smooth to touch, and shines in light. Diamond with six angles and facets are considered the best. The diamonds, which are spherical, dirty, bluish, or gray with lines, rough, and have physical defects are discarded and not used for astrological purposes. These are used in ayurvedic oral preparations, after processing. If used as such it is said to cause backache, vitiation of blood, hypothermia, chronic skin disease (leprosy), hallucination and sub-consciousness.

Astrologically diamond is connected with the planet Venus. It rules over throat, eyes, kidney and reproductive system. It increases attractiveness, artistic quality, grace and charm. When Venus is weak one may be coarse, crude or aggressive.

PROCESSING OF DIAMOND

Diamond is processed in many ways but the easiest method is to pulverize it and add to it red sulphide of mercury, processed sulphur and processed arsenic. Triturate the whole mixture and heat it in a crucible and let it cool. Repeat this process of heating and cooling thirteen times.

In another method, diamond is wrapped in a cloth pouch and this pouch is immersed in the decoction of *kodorav* (*Paspalum scrobiculatum*) or *kulthi* (*Dolichos biflorus*) for 3-7 days, dried and treated with decoction again. After 20-25 such treatments, diamond breaks into smaller pieces, and finally turns into a powder. It is processed further with *hartal* (arsenic compound), sulphur, *hingul* (arsenic compound), *Suvarnmakshik bhasam* (processed iron pyrite), one after the other and is macerated with the pulp of *Zizyphus* fruit. In the next step, whole mass is moistened with a decoction of *Ficus religiosa* to form a ball. This ball stored in a closed crucible is incinerated, cooled and heated again. This process of heating and cooling is repeated one hundred times.

Diamond may be processed by heating it to a high temperature and then dipping it in mercury. This treatment is repeated one hundred times. Diamond in this way breaks into small pieces after 20-25 treatments and finally turns into a fine powder.

THERAPEUTIC USES

Diamond processed by the above methods is said to be as good as *Amrita* (nectar) as it possess all the six desired virtues (*shad ras yukt*) required in a perfect Ayurvedic medicaments. It is as effective as mercurials as a therapeutic agent. It is considered a good *Rasayana* for cancer, tuberculosis, diabetes, and hepatotoxicity. It pacifies the inflammation of the digestive system, liver; helps in impotence by providing strength to the body. It is a geriatric cardiotonic, cerebral tonic, improves vision, and pacifies all the three *doshas*.

The dose in all the above cases is 2-4 mg depending on the condition of the patient

The processed diamond may also be used as follows:

Triturate 60 mg of processed diamond and 4 gm of red sulfide of mercury, till a uniform mixture is formed. Use a dose of 60-120 mg, with fresh milk- fat, *malai* (It is not butter but scum on top of fresh boiled milk. When milk is boiled, milk fat along with some proteinaceous materials come on the top, which on cooling forms a scum like layer, called *malai* which can be easily separated).

This preparation cures impotence and increases amorous power tremendously. It rejuvenates the body to such an extent that a man becomes sex-god (*kamdeva*) with pleasant personality, lustrous skin, sharp memory and immense physical strength. It also helps in chronic and obstinate cases of tuberculosis.

Sometimes instead of above preparation, processed diamond is used along with gold foil or in the following ways:

1. Mixed with *Makardhawaj* (red sulphide of mercury with gold) and administered in impotence.

Processed diamond mixed with camphor, sugar, cardamom seed, when administered with sweetened milk, if used for six months, provides immense sexual power to man to satisfy multiple partners. It makes man intelligent and as strong as a tiger.

Note: **In the above preparations diamond appears to** be a catalytic agent only as it is used with arsenic and mercury, which have profound physiological effect on the body.

G3 EMERALD *(Panna)*

It consists of silicate and oxides of aluminum, chromium and beryllium. Green colour of the stone is due to chromium oxide. Its hardness is 7.5, specific gravity 2.7-.8, and refractive index 1.57.

It is connected with the planet Mercury. It rules over the central nervous system, lungs and skin. It is said to give mental alertness, memory, communication skills, discriminative intellect, mental control and strength to the body. It detoxifies negativity, transforming it into positive energy. It is processed and used in the same way as ruby. Doze 30-120 mg

G4 FLOURSPAR or FLUORITE (*Vikrant*)

Chemically it is calcium fluoride. It is crystalline, has eight angles, with eight facets. It may be multicoloured, white, red, black or blue etc. The black variety is used in medicine.

There is a difference of opinion about the proper identification of *vikrant*. Some scholar postulate that it is a form of diamond.

For patients it acts as panacea whereas for healthy people it is a good *Rasayana*. In chronic and prolonged fevers it pacifies *tridosha prakopa*. It fortifies the effects of other medications. It is a geriatric tonic in wasting diseases, and incurable cases. It imparts immunity and develops resistance against diseases in healthy body. Doze: 5-10 mg

G5 GARNET or HESSONITE or AGATE (*Gomed*)

It is the gem for the planet *Rahu* of Indian astrology. Its colour is like that of cow's urine but has red lines. It is lustrous and beautiful with hardness of 7 to 7.5, specific gravity 3.65, and refractive index 1.74.

For medicinal use, it is roasted in lime-juice for three hours, then heated and processed. It pacifies *pitta.* It is an appetizer, increases the secretion of the digestive juices, cures all skin diseases and is a tonic for nervous system. It increases intellect and memory, and improves personality. It aids a sense of clarity and causes spiritual awakening Doze 30-125 mg

In *Siddha* System of Medicine, the stone opal is considered *Gomed*

G6 Glass Beads

(*Saphatika, Billore)*

It is natural, round, glass bead, rice- starch like in color. It is processed like *lajward.*

It has a cooling effect and it strengthens the body. It is anti-inflammatory in nature

G7 MOONSTONE or FELDSPAR or FELSPAR (*Lajward*)

It may be blue, gray, peach or even white but in Ayurveda the stone with blue hue, clear sky like smooth colour is preferred. Its hardness is 6

This stone is connected with moon. It rules over the blood and stomach and influences an individual's mind. Before use it is boiled in cow's urine, lime/lemon juice, natural potassium carbonate (*yavakshar*) for three hours in a closed vessel.

It helps in digestion, and in obesity and pacifies *pitta prakopa*

G8 RUBY *(Lal, Manikya)*

In India, ruby is commonly known as *lal* (red) but other names of this stone: *manikya, rangmanya, padamraj* and sunstone are frequently mentioned in literature. Ruby, which is blood red in colour, lustrous, cylindrical and uniform in structure is considered the best. It is made up of corundum and has hardness of 9, specific gravity 4, refractive index 1.76 and is composed of aluminum trioxide. It contains three elements: aluminum, iron and chromium.

Astrologically it is linked with sun, and was used by royality to focus and sustain their ability to command and rule. It sustains vitality and will. It enhances leadership, independence and purity. It affects heart, eyes and the bone system

In Ayurveda, it is used as a paste (*pishti*) or in calcined form (*bhasam*).

The paste can be prepared by triturating pulverized ruby in sandal water (water extract of wood of *Santalum album*), rose water (distillate of rose flower) and *kewra* water (distillate of *Pandanus odoratissmus* flower) and then heating it on mica.

For calcination, ruby is first purified by boiling it in an acidic fruit- juice. It is pulverized and triturated with equal quantities of purified sulphur, *Manshil*, (49 parts arsenic, 16 parts sulphur), *Hartal* (49 parts arsenic, 24 parts sulphur) and lemon juice. This mixture is dried in the sun for seven days, and heated in a crucible eight times.

The powdered ruby is considered a *Rasayana,* a brain tonic, and is given for strengthening the generative organs. It pacifies *kaph- prokopa*, and the other wasting diseases. It lubricates the body systems also.

For impotence, loss of semen and for heart- troubles, it may be taken in dose of 65-125 mg with milk cream once or twice a day or with gold foil with half teaspoon of honey twice a day.

Manikya Meheroday is a well known preparation of ruby. It is processed by mixing one part each of processed ruby, gold, silver, emerald, and two parts of musk. Whole mass is macerated in aloe pulp, and pills of 250 mg are made. It is considered an excellent *Rasayana*

G9 SAPPHIRE (*Neelam, Neel*)

In commerce sapphire of many colours are identified but in Ayurveda only blue colour (*neelam*) is used. In Astrology it is connected with the planet Saturn. It rules over the teeth, feet, bone, knees and nails. It helps bring balanced detachment, calm, and endurance. Sapphire is made up of corborundum and has hardness 9, specific gravity 3.97 to 4.0l and refractive index l.76.

This gem is purified by boiling it in the decoction of *Indigofera tinctoria*, and is processed like ruby. The product so obtained acts as an energizer, suppresses *tridosha,* lightens the skin color and is antidote to poisons. Dose 15-60 mg

In Indian trade, aquamarine, because of its sky blue colour, and amethyst, which is blue to violet in shade, is often used in place of sapphire

G10 SERPENTINE (*Zahar Mohra*)

Chemically it is magnesium silicate and is considered as an antidote to poisons.

RECENT STUDIES

JAWAHAR MOHRA (Ahmad *et al.* 1998)

Ingredients: Serpentine, lapis lazuli, jasper, agate, gum of *Vateria indica* and fruit of *Lodicea seychellarum* Labil.

This preparation was tried as an antistress agent against physical, chemical and metabolic stimuli. Results were encouraging.

G 11 SUNSTONE or BELAS RUBY or SPINAL RUBY or LENS (*Suryakant* or *Suryamani*)

It is spherical, transparent, convex lens like structure. It focus rays at one point. It may be pink, red, or may have other colours. It is transparent, soft to touch and lustrous. Its hardness is 5.5-8, specific gravity 2.5-3.6, and refractive-index is 1.72.

It has a *Rasayana* like effect particularly for brain and for *prakopa* of *pitta* and *kapha*. It is processed by pulverising it into fine powder and adding to it equal quantities of *manshil* (arsenic compound) and purified sulphur in a crucible. The mixture is heated and cooled seven times.

(Note: One more gem *Chanderkant* or *Chandermani* (moon gem) could not be identified but this is processed and used as *Suryamani*)

G12 TOPAZ (*Pushapraj, Pukhraj*)

This stone is yellow to orange in colour, transparent, and is often confused with citrine or yellow sapphire. It is a mixture of oxide of aluminum and oxy-fluoride of silicone. It has hardness of 8, specific gravity 3.5-3.53, and refractive index 1.61-1.64. When rubbed on other stones, clarity of this stone increases.

Astrologically it enhances the quality of planet Jupiter, such as wisdom, judgement, compassion, joyfulness, enthusiasm and faith.

In Ayurveda, it is purified by boiling it in *Dolichos biflorus* seed decoction, water extract of fermented cereals and is processed like ruby.

It is considered cooling in effect. It promotes digestive process, pacifies *kapha, vata*, cures leprosy and other skin diseases. It is antidote to poisons and has an antiinflammatory effect. If used by a healthy person, it acts as brain tonic, and helps in muscle building and longevity. It balances energy flow through the central nervous system, and helps in the alignment of body, mind and emotions

Dose 15-60 mg.

G13 TOURMALINE, PERIDOTE (*Panna bhed*)

Because of various shades of the green colour, peridote and tourmaline may be used in place of emerald. These stones are purified by washing them with milk and are calcined like ruby.

These are energizer, antidote to poison, digestant, form aura around the body and provide energy to the generative organs. These help in respiratory troubles, heart problems, deterioration of senses and in excessive fear. Dose: 15-60 mg

G14 TURQUOISE (*Firoza, Phiroza*)

It is bluish or ash colored stone, and is used as a fine paste by macerating it with sulphur, lime-juice for three days and then drying the whole mass in the sun.

It aids digestion, and is antidote to poisons.

REFERENCES FOR GEMS

Ahmad, G., Yusuf Amin, Khan, K.M., Tajuddin, N.A. (1998) The anti-stress activity of a gem containing Unani formulation against diverse stressors. *Journal of Ethnopharmacology*, **59**: 187-193.

Dash, V.B. *Alchemy and Metallic Medicines in Ayurveda*. Concept Pub., New Delhi (India).

Dash, V.B., Kashyap, V.L. *Iatro-chemistry of Ayurveda (Rasa Sastra).* Concept Pub., New Delhi (India).

Hodgson, Nick (through internet) Gems and Ayurveda.

Johri, Harish (1988) *Healing Power of Gem stones.in Tantra, Ayurveda and Astrology*. Destiny Books, Vermont (USA)

Kashinath Shastrina (1994) *Rastrangani* (in Hindi) 11th edition. Moti Lal Banarsi Das, Varanasi (India)

Kulkarni, P.H. (1998) *Ayurveda Minerals*. Indian Books Center, New Delhi

Nadkarni, K.M. (1954) *Indian Materia Medica*. Volume II, Popular Book Depot, Bombay (India).

Puri, H.S. (2003) RASAYANA: *Ayurvedic Herbs for Longevity and Rejuvenation*. Taylor & Francis, London, New York

Stein, Diane (2000) *Healing with Gemstones and Crystals*. Indian Book Center, New Delhi

ANIMAL PRODUCTS

INTRODUCTION

In Ayurveda, animals are broadly classified into two categories *Jangla* (terrestrial) and *Anupa* (aquatic).

JANGLA

This term was used generally for all types of the terrestrial animals, especially for the birds, wild- terrestrial reptiles and herbivorous mammals, on the basis of their living habitats. These included the following:

Reptiles and Mammals

1. *Vilastha*: those living under the ground such as amphibians, reptiles etc.
2. *Guhasaya*: carnivorous like tiger, lion, bear etc.
3. *Parnamriga*: arboreal such as monkey, squirrel etc.
4. *Gramya*: Domesticated animals like goat, cow etc.
5. *Jangla*: herbivorous like deer, stag etc.

Birds

1. *Vishkira*: birds like fowl, peacock, quail, which pick the food after scattering it.
2. *Pratuda*: birds like pigeon, which strike directly on the food
3. *Prasha*: Carnivorous birds like eagle, falcon etc.

ANUPA

This included hygrophytic and hydrophytic animals and were classified as:

Kulechara-those living in marshland such as buffalo, rhinoceros etc.

Plava- birds which swim on water such as ducks, cranes etc.

Kosastha- mollusc

Matsya – fish

Coral and pearl, which are parts of marine animals were considered minerals, and hence are not included in the above classification.

In ancient India, the flesh of many herbivorous animals, fish and birds was consumed as a general article of diet. From nutrition point of view flesh of *jangla*, *gramya* herbivorous animals and *vishkira* birds was preferred

The flesh and body parts of various animals were used for therapeutic purposes also, based on their supposed good effects on the body, as per the Ayurvedic principles, but a few *Rasayana* preparations in classical Ayurvedic texts contained animal flesh. In erotic literature of medieval India, *Kamasutra* and *Rati Rhasay* testes of goat and sheep have been prescribed. In one preparation testicles are to be boiled in milk, and sugar. In another sesame seed was added to this recipe. These were prescribed for vitality and virility in the body, which indicated that the sages at the time were aware of hormonal therapy.

Fresh animal parts like blood, flesh or eggs, were included in the Ayurvedic formulations to a limited extent but secondary animal products like honey, milk, butter, bones, molluscs, coral, pearl, musk, civet, ambergris and gall bladder (dry) etc. both from terrestrial and marine animals were extensively used. As a medium of administration for medications, the use of fluid nutrients like honey, milk and milk products and *ghee* was very much advocated.

Cow has a very important place in Indian culture and is worshipped by Hindus even now. Consequently anything obtained from cow has a great sentimental value in Hindu psyche. A product *Panchgavya,* made by mixing cow's urine, cow's dung, milk, yogurt and *ghee* is sometimes considered a panacea. Many recipes of milk, yogurt and *ghee* are also used for longevity. According to one postulation, any one or all of these i.e., water kept overnight in clay pot, fresh milk, pure honey and cow's *ghee*, have cooling (*sheetal*) effect and should be consumed by the person who is suffering from diseases originated due to excessive heat in the body.

In the following pages, detail about the animals, animal by products or animal parts, which are ingredient of many *Rasayana* preparations, is given.

TERRESTRIAL ANIMAL S

A1 BUTTER (*Makhan*)

Butter obtained after churning yogurt is easy to digest and causes general development of the body. Only fresh butter should be used, on storage it becomes sour, which causes gastric upsets and is not safe to use. The fresh butter increases sexual power, helps in gastro-enteritis, *vayu pitta*, *rakta pitta*, piles and cough. It lubricates intestinal canal, makes skin attractive and fresh. Butter obtained from cow's milk is considered the best but that from goat milk considered more powerful. Butter obtained from buffalo milk is a bit hard to digest

Butter obtained by churning yogurt made from the milk in which *Calotropis* flowers, *Nerium indicum* root and ginger have been boiled, is used as nervine tonic and as an aphrodisiac. For use, small quantity of this butter is smeared on the betel leaves.

Butter, *ghee* and other milk products are given as per the digestive power of the patient. To avoid any side effects *Triphala* (a mixture of equal quantities of the dry fruits of *Emblica oficinalis, Terminalia bellerica* and *T. chebula*) is administered along with.

It consists of largely of butter fat, which is made up of stearin. Butyric, palmitic and oleic acids are the fatty acids found in butter fat.

A2 BUTTER OIL (*Ghrit, Ghee*)

It is prepared by heating butter to remove moisture and non-fatty matters to get anhydrous butter fat. In this way the butter has a very good keeping quality, and can be stored for years together. It is also called clarified butter and in Latin *butyrum depurarum* but clarified butter as used in French and South American cuisine, during its preparation it is cooked for shorter time, and thus all of the water and solids are not removed. In Indian sub-continent in the last century, another product made by hydrogenation of fatty oils (like margarine), has also been introduced, which mainly consist of trans fatty acids but is very much like *ghee* in appearance and action. To distinguish the two the *ghee* obtained from butter is commonly called *desi ghee* or *asli ghee* and that from oils as vegetable *ghee*. Earlier it was mandatory in India to add sesame oil to vegetable *ghee* so that it may be distinguished from the real *ghee* by simple chemical tests but no such restriction is there now and any oil can be used for hydrogenation. Another form of vegetable *ghee* is prepared by mixing palm oil and soybean oil or sometimes *ghee* is totally or partially substituted by animal fats. Whereas hydrogenated oil and *ghee* can be distinguished by exposing them to ultra-violet light, where the catalyst used in hydrogenated oil gives characteristic fluorescence, it is not possible to detect the other type of adulterations from *ghee* easily.

In India, three methods are used for preparation of *ghee* from butter. These are:

1. Heat butter in a container. The butter for this is obtained, by subjecting milk to mechanical processes (centrifugal separators) so that the fat containing cream, which is lighter, get separated from the rest of milk This cream is cultured to obtain butter.

2. Remove the scum (*malai*), which appears as top layer after boiling and cooling milk. Macerate this scum and get *ghee* by heating it.

3. Prepare yogurt from the whole milk, when yogurt is ready, in the morning, add water to it and churn it vigorously so that the butter separates from the diluted liquid yogurt as a lump on the top. Heat this butter to get the *ghee*. It is also known as *Loni* or *Noni ghee* and is considered the best.

Recent studies have shown that when milk is subjected to vigorous churning by machines, as in the case of first method, then only a very small quantity of unsaturated fatty acid linolenic acid gets separated from the milk, hence the *ghee* prepared in this way, as is the case of most of the commercial products, has a small quantity of this acid, whereas the ghee prepared in the third way, which is not subjected to strong mechanical force, has much larger quantity of this acid. That is why the *ghee* obtained from the butter prepared in traditional way has more nutritive property as compared to the one prepared by the modern machines. In the traditional way milk is subjected to low heat and low mechanical force, which help in the extraction of maximum amount of unsaturated fatty acids from the milk.

In all these three methods, butter on slow heating gets converted into two fractions: liquid and solid. While warm, the liquid fraction is removed by filtering through muslin or cheese- cloth, which on cooling gets solidified. The product so obtained is called *ghee*.

Ghee in the case of cow's milk is pale yellowish in colour with a very pleasant smell and taste and is considered the best. The milk of other animals is also utilized for this purpose. The *ghee* obtained from the animals other than the cow has the following Ayurvedic qualities:

Buffalo: Hard to digest, produces *kaph* in the body but balances *vata* and *pitta*. It detoxifies the blood.

Goat: Digestant, invigourates the body, clears vision and helps in respiratory diseases.

Sheep: Digestant, strengthens the bone and helps in kidney stone and diabetes.

Sometimes before incorporation in the medicine *ghee* is repeatedly washed by pouring fresh water on it and rubbing it with hands. After every wash the old water is thrown and the fresh water is added. The process is repeated twenty one times to remove all the water- soluble constituents.

In Ayurveda, fresh *ghee* is considered an item of food and is incorporated in all types of daily diets but when one year old it is used for medicinal purposes only. Older the ghee better it is in its effect. Some scholar consider one year old *ghee* as old enough while the other maintain that it should be at least ten years old. The ghee, which is eleven years old is called, "*kumbhisarp*" and hundred year old as "*kronch*". There is mention of more than thousand years old as *Mahaghrit* but it appears hypothetical as no body has any record for it since antiquity.

THERAPEUTIC USES IN AYURVEDA AND FOLK-LORE

Ghee is a *Rasayana,* anti *pitta*, anti *kapha* and anti *vata*, cooling in nature. It is base of a number of Ayurvedic preparations called *ghritam* or *ghrit* as it one of the very few fats or oils which remain stable at higher temperature. In these preparations fresh herbs or the decoctions of dry herbs are heated with *ghee* till no water is left. The medicated *ghee* is filtered through cloth and used. In these preparations, *ghee* extracts all the fat soluble constituents of the herb, which in a very low concentration help the body. *Brahmi ghrit* made with *Centella asiatica* and other herbs, *Nimba ghrit,* and *Panch tikatam ghrit* made from *Azadirachta indica*, are some of the well known preparations.

Ghee is slightly heavy to digest, but improves strength, personality, brain, aura, beauty, intelligence, and memory, particularly in old age. If it is being given along with some medicaments, it should be consumed as per the digestive power of the patient. The people with week constitution should take two tea spoonful *ghee* with equal quantity of sugar, till there is no digestive problem. If there is uneasiness, the dose may be reduced or stopped. Common symptoms of over consumption of *ghee* are, diarrhoea, indigestion and heaviness in the stomach.

It is mainly used for the following purposes:

In nose bleeding

Drop a few drops of molten *ghee* in the nostril twice daily, for a couple of days till cured.

In piles

In hemorrhoids where there is a discharge of blood,

mix one teaspoon full each of *ghee*, sesame seed and sugar candy (*mishri*) and take thrice daily.

In headache

In sudden flaring of the symptoms, massage the sole of the feet with *ghee* for three or four days.

For improving the eye-sight

Eat sugar candy (*mishri*) with *ghee*.

In night blindness

Make a decoction of one teaspoon full of *triphala* (equal parts of fruits of *Emblica officinalis*, *Terminalia bellerica* and *Terminalia chebula*). Mix one tea spoon *ghee* in it and drink.

As antidote to poisons

When used in small quantities it removes inert undesirable constituents from food. It also acts as a blood purifier in the case of vitiation of blood. In *Datura* and mercury poisoning it acts as antidote to these poisons. In the case of other poisons and snake- bite, give to the victim about125 gm *ghee*. The patient will vomit the poison out.

In unconsciousness

Administration of ten years old *ghee* and massage of it on the forehead helps. *Ghee* when mixed with the herb *Alhagi camelorum* is also effective.

As an immunostimulant

It enhances immunity in the body to fight various diseases. As per Ayurveda, it plays a good role in stabilizing metabolism in the body by pacifying all the three *doshas* and increasing all the seven *dhatus*.

As a nutrient

It extracts fat- soluble vitamin A, D, and E from our foods and makes them available to the body. If we use *ghee* we may not need these additional vitamin supplements.

It is of particular importance for athletes and those indulging in heavy physical labour. It is slightly heavy to digest, but improves strength, personality, brain, aura, beauty, intelligence, and memory, particularly in old age.

As an anti-cancerous agent

It probably makes inert the cancer causing agents in the body. This effect probably is due to linolenic acid contained in it.

In nervous diseases

It improves eye-sight. It helps in hysteria, migraine, schizophrenia and unconsciousness.

As a laxative

It acts as a lubricator in constipation.

In hiccough

In the case of hiccough ingestion of worm *ghee* helps

As an antacid

Whereas fatty oil leads to the production of acidity in the body, *ghee* is antacid.

As an air purifier

The fumigants of *ghee* is said to have an antimicrobial

effect that is why *ghee* lamp is used in religious gatherings, in *havan-* ceremony and during cremation of dead bodies.

For skin diseases

Ghee is much esteemed for application over wounds, inflammation, swellings, blisters and for promotion of quick healing. It can be safely used as an ear- drop, nasal-drop, and for face to improve complexion and impart beauty.

For external use an ointment from *ghee* is made by repeatedly washing it in a brass utensil, sometimes 100 times or even more. In this way *ghee* becomes poisonous, probably by contamination with copper and zinc and should be used for skin diseases only.

For covering the burns

It can be used in place of sesame oil for application on burns.

In cracking of the soles of the feet

A mixture of salt and *ghee* softens the skin. In winter it helps the dry skin.

As an anti-allergic agent

For quick healing, *ghee* is dropped into nostril in coryza. For air borne allergens *ghee* smeared inside the nostril or instilled in nasal canal, acts as an anti-inflammatory agent. The effect may be due to formation of a protective cover over the mucus membrane of the nostril.

In gynecological practice

As a source of vitamin D, it helps in osteomalacia, during pregnancy. It also provides required nutrition to foetus and mother and assures normal delivery. It is customary in India to give a diet high in *ghee* during pre natal and post natal period.

In bronchial problems

A mixture of *ghee* and rock salt is massaged on the chest. Warm *ghee* helps in hiccough also.

In arteriosclerosis

When used in moderate quantities, *ghee* actually protects against arteriosclerosis, as heart-diseases are triggered due to eating of processed carbohydrates and fats.

In alcoholism

When two- teaspoon full *ghee* with equal quantity of sugar are administered to a drunkard, it helps. The mixture shows its effect even after heavy drinking.

RECENT STUDIES

Ghee is very rich in saturated fatty acids, and cholesterol oxide, which increase serum total cholesterol in human body and causes changes in arterial structure leading to atherosclerosis. A large volume of study substantiates this observation and people are advised not to use *ghee* in their daily diet. On the other hand Dr Raheja of All India Institute of Diabetes, Bombay, as quoted by Bala (1999) said that in chasing the phantom of cholesterol, it (*ghee*) was condemned as highly saturated fat believing that the lower consumption of it lowered the risk of heart attack but it proved otherwise. Large contents of palmitic acid and myristic acid in it effect some anti-diabetogenic action as they stimulate glucose mediated insulin secretions and thus help in the cardio-vascular diseases.

According to a modern concept, for leak proof cell membrane of the brain, fatty oils with *cis*-configuration form are required, which are mostly obtained from unprocessed fats. *Ghee* may be providing these required essential fatty acids as most of the present day edible fats and oils are processed by heating them at high temperature, and/ or by hydrogenation, bleaching and deodorizing. These activities destroy *cis* configuration of the fatty acids. The brain cannot use this form and hence brain cell membrane gets leaked if only these fatty acids are used.

Due to the presence of phytoestrogens, antioxidants and other constituents, *ghee* blocks the absorption of other fats into the blood and hence reduces cholesterol. It also contains polyphenolic compounds which stimulate nitric oxide levels and reduce high blood pressure. The *ghee* phytosterols also inhibit cholesterol absorption and may suppress colon cancer and prostate cancer by interfering with steroid hormone production.

DETECTION OF ADULTERATION

It is often adulterated or substituted by hydrogenated oils (*vanaspati ghee*), animal fats, palm oil and other edible oils. Sometimes potato or sweat potato, starch of which gets gelatinized on prolonged boiling is also mixed in it.

As mentioned earlier, any adulteration in *ghee* even in minutest quantities can be easily detected by observing the fluorescence emitted by it, by placing it under ultra-violet lamps. Gelatinized starch in *ghee* can be detected by simple iodine test. If there is any starch it will turn black, otherwise the iodine reagent remains dark brown.

Hydrogenated oils, which are very much like *ghee*, are the common adulterants but are hard to detect in a rural set up, so in these area, the common test is differential behaviour of pure and adulterated *ghee* in mustard oil. Pure ghee settles at the bottom of mustard oil whereas *vanaspati ghee* floats in it. An other simple test is performed by smearing *ghee* on the outer surface of an earthen pitcher and observing it for some time. Pure *ghee* is absorbed by clay but any adulteration is left behind on the surface of clay as a white layer.

CONTRAINDICATION

Ghee should not be administered to infant, aged, obese or to weak persons, or to patients of tuberculosis, respiratory problem, cholera, and indigestion. *Ghee* shows its beneficial effects only after digestion, if it remains undigested in the body, it may create many metabolic disturbances, so should be consumed only in limited quantity. The young, the old and the person who do not have much physical activity cannot digest it and should consume the *ghee* and its products in a very limited amount.

REFERENCES

Al-Khalifa, A and Al-Khatani (1993) Composition of ghee (Samn Barri) from cow's milk and sheep milk. *Food Chemistry* **46**:373-375

Bala Murali Krishna (1999) Coconut oil, ghee check diabetes. *The Times of India* 12/15/1999

Feldenkreis, Kathyrn, S. (1996) *Ghee: A guide to the Royal oil*. Morris Publishing

Jacobson, M.S. (1987) Cholesterol oxide in Indian Ghee: possible cause of unexplained high risk of atherosclerosis in Indian immigrant population. *Lancet*, **2(8560)**: 656-658.

Prasad, Lallan Kumar (2003) Ghee (in Hindi) *Health and Nutrition (India)* 60-63

Pritechford, P. (1993) *Healing with Whole Foods*. North Atlantic Books, Berekley.

Singh, R.B. (1196) Association of trans fatty acids (vegetable ghee) and clarified butter (Indian ghee) intake with higher rise of coronary artery diseases in rural and urban population with low fat consumption. *Journal of Cardiology*, **56**: 289-298

A3 CASTOREUM (*Jundbedstar*)

It is obtained from a squirrel like animal, a beaver (*Castor* spp., class Rodentia), who has flat scaly tail, and pair of gland in anal region (preputial follicle) that secret an oil, which gets collected in the pockets in this area. These pouches are brownish in colour, about 8 cm long, full of solid brown or black concrete secretion with a unique musk like odour. In some cases, it has a strong unpleasant odour, an acidic bitter taste resembling that of cat's urine.

The concretion is commonly known as *Jundbedstar* in India, and is used in place of musk but is weaker in action. It is said to have a strong stimulant effect on the nervous system, particularly on the generative organs of the females. It is often prescribed in hysteria, epilepsy, amenorrhoea, dysmenorrhoea, and as massage oil for males. A supreme aphrodisiac preparation is prepared by macerating *Jundbedsatr* in honey, musk, and spices and is administered after wrapping it in gold and silver foils.

A4 CIVET CAT (*Jabad Kasturi*)

This animal *Viveria zibetha* (civet cat) resembles a cat but has a longer tail, and black spots on the body. It is found in south India and in some parts of south Asia and Africa. The animal has a pouch divided into two parts between anal region and penis. The pouch contains civet of commerce, which is extracted by trapping the animals in small, narrow cage and squeezing the civet out of the pouch. In its natural form the smell of civet is strong and penetrating, but after treatment and mixing it with other inert substances, the smell becomes mild and musk like.

In Malabar (south India) the farmer erect bamboo in their farms, the animal masturbates with this bamboo, and the dry spermatic fluid, dark in colour, is collected and is known as *Punnugu* or *Jabadi*. It may be an admixture of small twigs, hair, etc.

In Bengal (east India) the scrotum sac of testicles, area surrounding the pouch and spermatic fluid of this cat is dried and sold as *khattashi*, which imparts pleasant aroma to a massage oil *Naryana tail*, which not only increases pleasure during sexual intercourse but acts as an antifertility agent also. *Khattashi* is often adulterated with other materials.

Civet is considered hot in nature, aromatic, stimulant, antiinflammatory, nervine tonic, and aphrodisiac. The alcoholic extract helps in depression and heart palpitation. Civet and saffron with chicken soup facilitates delivery. In migraine and headache its smell helps. When mixed in almond oil and dropped in ear, it increases the hearing power.

A5 EGG (*Dimb, Andey*)

The eggs from various birds are considered a good aphrodisiac, spermatogentic, and nourishing. These are said to impart strength, pacify *vata* and are considered useful in loss of virility

Outer shell of the egg, which is very rich in calcium, is commonly used as a nutritive, as a source of calcium, but is processed before use.

EGG -SHELL *Bhasam*

It is prepared by keeping egg- shell in a mixture of water and salt for about 12 hours. After this the shell is dried and pulverized. The powder so obtained is mixed with lemon juice or aloe pulp and heated for 12 hours. This process of heating is repeated for seven times.

Five gm of this processed shell with honey or butter is administered in leucorrhoea, enlargement of liver and spleen, and for flatulence.

A6 FAT (*Vasa, Charbi*)

In addition to their high calorific value as food, the fats from animals have a strong penetrating powers in the skin, so are used as a medium for massage ointments to strengthen the muscles, as in the case of aches of pains and those of the sexual organs. Earlier fat from the body of carnivorous animals like tiger, bear was used in a number of preparations. If these fats were not available then they were substituted by that from the wild boar but now these fats are used only to a very limited extent in remote areas. Sometimes fat obtained from the eggs as such or with arsenic, is used.

The well known fat for massage, is from a lizard like animal, known as *Sanda* (*Gecko verticillatus*, *Iguana*). The fat is obtained by boiling the animal in water. On cooling the fat being lighter than water, comes on the top. It is collected and is sold as oil of *Sanda*.

A7 FLESH (*Mans*)

As per the old Ayurvedic texts, the terrestrial animals and birds are called *Jangla jeev*. The flesh of these animals is considered anabolic, vitaliser and good for *tridosha*. Out of these flesh of goat is preferred and is considered demulcent, nutritious, cardiac stimulant, and generative of semen. Flesh of peacock (*mor*) and partridge (*tittar*) gets easily digested and is good for sick and convalescent. The flesh of partridge is also a cardiac stimulant, improves memory and alleviates *tridosha*, while that of pigeon and peacock is good nutritive and improves memory. In some areas of south India, dried flesh of tiger/lion is given to young children to impart bravery in them.

In Ayurveda, two preparations, *Hansadi Ghrit* from flesh of geese and *Chagaladi ghrit* from goat flesh are used as nervine tonic in cephalalgia and nervous diseases. Both products are prepared in the same way.

The *Chagaladi ghrit* is prepared by boiling together goat meat 6.250 kg, ten herbs *Dasmula* 6.250 kg, and water 64 liter, till the water is reduced to about one fourth. The soup so obtained is filtered. In an other container this soup and 4 kg each of *ghee*, milk, juice/decoction of *shatawari* (*Asparagus racemosus*), and a herbal paste 1 kg made from *Gaduchi* (*Tinospora cordifolia*), *banslochan* (bamboo manna), *ashwagandha* (*Withania somnifera*), *anantmul* (*Hemidesmus indicus*), *kakoli* (*Curculigo orchioides*), *ksheerkakaoli* (*Chlorophytum arundinaceum*), beans (*Phaseolus trilobus* and *Glycine debilis*), *jivanti* (an orchid) and liquorice root are boiled together till all water evaporates and only ghee is left

Uses: For various nervous diseases, facial paralysis, convulsion, hysteria, sciatica etc.

Another preparation, *Masha Taila* is prepared by boiling 8 kg goat meat in 64 kg of water in a container, till water is reduced to one fourth. In an other container, 1 kg each of *Phaseolus roxburghii*, linseed, barley, root of *Barleria prionitis*, *Solanum jacquinii*, *Tribulus terrestris*, Oroxylum *indicum Nardostachys jatamansi, and Mucuna pruriens* seed are boiled in 64 liter of water, till water is reduced to one fourth In a third container, 2 kg each of the seed of cotton, *Crotalaria juncea*, *Dolichos biflorus*, dried pulp of *Zizyphus jujuba*, are boiled in 64 liter of water till it is reduced to one fourth. A paste from 1 kg mixture of equal parts of ginger, long peppr, dill, root of *Ricinus communis*, *Boerhaavia diffusa*, *Paederia foetida*, *Vanda roxburghii* (*rasna*) *Sida cordifolia*, *Tinospora cordifolia*, and *Picrorrhiza kurroa*, is made. All the three decoctions, obtained above are filtered, mixed together along with the paste and boiled in 4 kg sesame oil till no water is left in the mixture.

This oil is used for external application along with *Chagaladi ghrit*

A8 HONEY (*Madhu, Shahad*)

In Mesopotamia, where civilization is believed to have begun in 5000 BC, honey was known. In addition to many other uses, the ancient Egyptian preserved dead bodies with honey. Indian yogis have always maintained that honey is a "spiritual" food, containing a special power to help to balance the body's life force energies.

The source of honey is nectar of the flowers, collected by the bees. The saccharose of the nectars is converted into invert sugars (dextrose and laevulose) in the honey- comb by the enzyme invertase, which is contained in the salivary secretion of bee. When a considerable amount of honey is deposited in the bee- hive, it is removed. The honey is separated from the cells of the honey- comb by cutting, draining and centrifuging or by pressure with or without the use of heat.

Honey obtained from different flowers and geographical regions varies in appearance. The colour and odour of honey differ according to place of their collection. If the flowers of a locality are poisonous so will be the honey of that area. In western countries clover honey is preferred where as that from coniferous forest or eucalyptus plantation because of the camphoraceous odour is considered inferior. Earlier in India, honey obtained from lotus flower growing in Kashmir, Bengal and Himalayas, was considered the best. This was called white honey or lotus honey. In south India, honey by small bees (it is probably a different species) in small hives is considered the best and that of bigger hives on big tree trunks, of inferior quantity.

Honey is dark brown to yellow, semi-liquid or a white crystalline mass, exhibiting plates of dextrose crystals under the microscope. Honey consists almost entirely of a concentrated watery solution of invert sugar (70%)) and small quantity of saccharose, dextrin and protein substances, colouring matter, formic and mallic acids, about 15% water, traces of mineral matter, volatile oil, proteolytic enzymes and gummy substances. It also has compound called phenolics that have antioxidant properties. It is acidic due to the presence of the organic acids.

Quite often fresh honey on keeping separates into two layers, the liquid upper and semi solid lower. Sometimes, viscosity of honey may increase on storage. It is a natural phenomenon. The liquid part of the honey consists of more of fruit sugar and less of grape sugar. This type of honey is good for diabetics. If honey separates in two physical forms in cold conditions, it can be made uniform by heating it slightly in hot water container. Once heated honey remains as a homogenous fluid so most of commercial products are treated this way before packing.

Fresh honey is preferred as an article of diet in most parts of India. Honey, which is malodorous, sour or bitter in taste, due to fermentation should be avoided. Usually 50 gm honey in five divided dozes is administered with water, fruit juices, milk etc., but it should not be prescribed to individuals with empty stomach in the morning, particularly to pregnant ladies, in hot climate or when there are symptoms of "heat" in the body. It should also not be taken with rain- water, sugar of any type, fatty oils and non-vegetarian diet. When mixed in cold milk, it has an anabolic effect and increases weight but with 1-3 spoon in cold water before passing stool in the morning, it dissolves fat from the body, if used for two months. If honey is to be mixed with *ghee* as a nutrient, never mix equal quantities of both as this mixture is said to have deleterious effect on the body. In this case four to five times honey with one part of *ghee* should be used.

According to Ayurveda, honey does not deteriorate in quality even after years of storage. On the other hand storage increases the therapeutic efficacy of honey. The old honey is said to be lighter, digests quickly and brings about digestion, is laxative and anti-obesity in nature. Fresh honey is a good nutritive and relieves the body from *vata* and *kapha.*

THERAPEUTIC USES

Honey is a household remedy in India, and used extensively. Recently it has been seen that it is not only a good natural sweetener but has phenolics, which have a good antioxidant properties. These phenolics quench free radicals, which are unstable byproducts of normal metabolism that cause damage to arteries and to DNA that can lead to cancer and other diseases.

The major uses of this product are:

For improving eye sight

Mix honey in carrot juice, drink this juice in the morning one hour before breakfast for 40 days in winter. It removes tension and improves vision.

For cataract

One drop of white honey when applied to the eye is

said to prevent cataract. When applied regularly, it cleans eyes, improves vision and relieves tension

As a mental tonic

Masticate thoroughly, 2-3 walnut kernels with 1-2 spoonful of honey in the morning.

As a cardiotonic

Mix one tea spoonful fennel powder with honey. It acts as a blood purifier also.

In bronchial troubles (*Kaph prakopa*)

Honey when mixed with ginger juice gives relief in bronchial problems. It is a good expectorant. If black pepper is added to the above mixture, it increases its effectiveness.

In weakness

As an anabolic agent in general weakness swallow 2-3 tea- spoonful of honey with the main meals or drink honey with cold milk, without sugar before sleep.

In high blood pressure

Crush 3-4 cloves in honey and chew the whole mixture.

As an anthelmintic

Mix one teaspoonful *neem* (*Azadirachta indica*) leaf juice with 2 3 tea-spoonful of honey for 3-4 days.

In cold and cough

Use one tea- spoonful noney, with 5-6 *tulsi* (*Ocimum sanctum*) leaves

As a blood purifier for skin diseases

In a glass full of water, squeeze one lemon/lime and add one tea spoonful of honey. Drink this mixture empty stomach in the morning.

For fatigue

One tea- spoonful of honey in a glass of water, provides immediate energy because of levulose and dextrose contained in it.

For small ulcers in the mouth

Crush 2-3 gm cardamom seeds, mix them in a tea-spoonful of honey and apply this mixture over the ulcers.

In nervous diseases

For sciatica and paralysis, honey water, which is prepared by boiling two parts of water with one part honey till one part of water remains, is used. Any scum, which appears during boiling is removed.

In diabetes

In the cases, where after medication or otherwise glucose level goes down suddenly, and may make the patient unconscious due to diminished brain function, honey restores sugar level in the body. Spoon for spoon, it is thought that honey contains 21% fewer calories than an equal amount of refined- sugar.

Carbohydrates in honey improved recovery in 39 well-trained athletes during the two hours following an intense weight lifting session. After a work out, an increase in insulin promoted metabolism and, lowered blood sugar levels but honey maintained an optimum level of blood sugar. It also created a good hormone ratio indicating that muscle recuperated quickly.

As a sedative

Warm milk with honey induces sleep

In pharmaceuticals

As a sweetening agent, it is used as vehicle for most of the products, which are not pleasant to taste. It acts as a demulcent and as preservative also. It increases the bioavailability of therapeutic agent so it is called '*yogavahi*'. It is added to some medications for increasing their shelf life. It is alleged that even a dead body can be nicely preserved if immersed in honey. In medieval India, it was a common practice to store perishable fruits, particularly mango for months, in honey.

For digestive system

Honey is particularly useful in malnutrition, convalescence, hepatotoxicity and in geriatric cases. It is not only a valuable diet, but also keeps digestive system in order. Its natural occurring mixture of simple and complex sugars, may allow for slower release of carbohydrates. It relieves constipation, provides strength to stomach and serves as a good appetizer. Rose water is said to enhance its effect. The person who cannot digest milk easily can do so easily by the addition of honey.

In gynecological practices

It is said to smoothen the flow during menstruation and helps during lactation. During pregnancy it is a good nutrient both for child and mother. It should not be used continuously throughout pregnancy twice daily, but with break from time to time. Use milk or fruit juice for diluting it. With the use of honey anemia, weakness etc are not seen. It helps in other gynoecological problems like leucorrhea and dysmenorrhea

For skin diseases

Externally honey with common salt and vinegar is used for clearing blemishes and the other spots from the body.

As an aphrodisiac

For men honey is a good tonic for all systems of the body, for all ages. It increases sexual power, gives strength to the body. For powerful, sexual act,· liquorice with mixture of honey and *ghee* with sweetened milk is given

As a mental tonic

It is a good mental tonic particularly for students. Soak almond in water, when soft make a paste and use this paste with honey. It should be used continuously for 40 days in all ages and stages. Honey gives relief in headache, sexual inadequacies, fatigue, tiredness, and acts as an immunostimulant.

For infants

Four to five drops of honey in one tea-spoonful of milk twice daily acts as a laxative, relives belching, keeps respiratory passage clear, helps in prevention of constipation, flatulence, bronchial problems and induces good sleep. As a vermifuge, it should be mixed with yogurt. During teething troubles make a paste of honey with crude borax and apply. Regular use of honey with milk makes body strong and healthy.

As a nutrient for women

It imparts health and beauty, when used 10 gm, twice daily for 40 days. After this give a break. Do not use honey continuously for months together. During pregnancy, for the health of new- born baby, use honey with a break, for a couple of days from time to time. It helps in anemia, general weakness in the body and insomnia. It makes the body healthy, charming and beautiful. It gives proper figure to weak women and slim figure in obesity. It adds fat to the body when used with cold milk but removes fat when used with cold water. Lean and thin girls should drink honey (10 gm) with cold milk (200 ml) for 40 days. Give a break for some days do not use continuously. Obese women should drink honey with water instead of milk as above

CONTRAINDICATION

Honey should not be used, if any toxic or side effects are observed with its usage. Do not use honey alone in empty stomach in the morning - it may cause gastric pain.

ADULTERATION

It is sometimes adulterated with water, starch sugar, cane sugar, artificial honey, dextrin, glycerine, synthetic honey perfume and colouring matter. These can be detected by simple chemical tests.

In Indian Pharmacopoeia, the following standards have been set for honey:

Weight per ml: should not be less than 0.36 gm

Acid value: not exceeding 0.5 ml N NaOH in 10 gm

Ash content: not to exceed 0.5%

A9 HORNS (*Shring, Seeng*)

Out of various herbivorous animals, stag horn along with antlers of other allied species are used in Ayurvedic medicines. The horn, which is not moth ridden or spongy but is hard and heavy is cut into small pieces by saw and is incinerated. The ash so obtained on cooling is macerated with the latex of *Calotropis.* The mass is made into small balls and incinerated again. The process is repeated two more times till grayish to white ash is obtained but gray ash is preferred. This ash is rich in calcium phosphate, and provides nutrient to the body. Sometimes instead of incineration, horn is made into a paste by rubbing it on the rough stone, and used.

These horn preparations are considered a restorative tonic, useful in respiratory and sexual problems. With *ghee,* the horn ash gives relief in acute angina pectoris and any type of pain in the pectoral region. In acute respiratory diseases, it is prescribed with *Zizyphus* kernel, *Achyranthes aspera* seed and long pepper. Dry black grapes and date palm fruits are said to enhance the effect of this preparation.

A10 LAC or SHELL LAC (*Lakh*)

It is a deep red or brown secretion of an insect *Laccifer lacca* on the branches of old trees. Lac from *Ficus religiosa*, collected in April-May is considered the best. It is collected and stored in a cloth- bag, the bag is subjected to heat by which filtered lac comes out of it, keeping the debris and vegetable matters in the bag.

In Ayurveda, lac is said to makes skin lustrous. It imparts strength to the body. It is anti-inflammatory in action, and is mainly used in oil *Chandan baladi-lakshadi tailam* for external application.

A11 LIZARD (*Reg Mahi*)

These are esteemed in Arab countries and became popular in India because of trade contacts. One of these. *Reg Mahi*, *Lacerta agilis* (*Agama agilis*) is sand lizard with thorny spine. After collection its head and legs are decapitated, and skin removed. On drying it appears like fish and many people confuse it with fish. It is light brown in colour with dark brown regulation on the back about 15 cm long. In India, the ash of this animal with yolk of egg is used as a nervine tonic, aphrodisiac and stimulant in spermatorrhoea and seminal weakness. In other countries the pulverized powder of the lizard is taken with sweet white wine. In Punjab (Indo-Pakistan) *Mabuia carinata* is also called *Reg Mahi*, the fat of this animal is used as aphrodisiac, restorative and stimulant. In some other areas another lizard *Sticus officinalis* is also used. A giant lizard like animal, Iguana may also be used for the same purpose.

A12 MILK (*Dugdh, Doodh*)

It is not only a complete food, but is the first food for most of the terrestrial mammals. All the herbivorous animals are good source of milk but in Ayurveda, mainly milk of mother, cow, buffalo and goat is used.

Cow's milk, preferably that of black one, is said to have the same quality as that of mother's milk (in the text wherever milk is mentioned, it means cow's milk). Buffalo milk with higher fat contents is hard to digest. Goat- which mainly grazes on leaves of trees of all types including bitter and astringent one, drinks less water and indulges in physical activity whole day, is said to yield a very nutritive milk, which helps in many diseases because of its antimicrobial properties. It is particularly given to the patients of tuberculosis.

As an article of diet, only warm milk, such as fresh milk direct from the animals, should be used. If this is not possible then boil stored milk and use it when warm. Cold milk should be avoided. Best time for drinking milk is about two hours, after dinner in the evening. It should be chewed and not swallowed. After boiling and while still warm, the fat of the milk comes as a scum (*malai*) on the top. The persons with good digestive power, should drink this whole milk, with this fat while in the other cases, milk fat may be removed.

Milk in Ayurveda is considered anti- *vata,* anti-*pitta*, spermatogenic (tissue builder), and aphrodisiac. It is cooling in its effect and provides strength and energy for longevity. It is particularly prescribed in high fevers, mental diseases, and as a cardiotonic in all types of weaknesses.

It is a supreme food, having cooling, nutritive, immunostimulant, brain tonic, geriatric tonic, vitalizer, spermatogenic and demulcent effects. It has been prescribed for most of *Rasayana* preparations as a medium of administration, and it is said to sustain life and helps in curing all types of diseases of the body. It should be used during all types of physical and mental activity, preferably after sexual intercourse.

In Ayurveda, for arsenic preparations, arsenic is boiled in milk for a long time at low temperature till it gets dissolved in milk. This evaporated, condensed milk in extremely low dozes is given for boosting immunity to the body in winter and in rainy season. The doze is increased steadily. Earlier this was mainly prescribed for malaria.

Milk contains L-carnitine, which is forerunner of many new neuroprotective compounds that can maintain brain.

In a study it was seen that the milk obtained for a few days after delivery of cow is rich in colostrum. Colostrum contain white blood cells, protective antibodies, protein and fat in a thin yellow liquid and helps in many intestinal diseases. It is anti-inflammatory and anti-ulcerative in action.

Milk, which has turned sour or has developed a different colour, bad taste, and smell or is stored for a longer period, should not be used.

Milk is contraindicated in respiratory and gastric diseases such as hyperacidity and flatulence.

A13 MUSK (*Kasturi*)

Musk is a strong smelling oleo-resin obtained from musk deer, which is an important ingredient of many high class perfumes even now.

In Ayurveda three type of musk has been recognized. These are: from alpine Kashmir (western Himalayas), Nepal (central Himalayas) and Kamrup (Arunachal, eastern Himalayas). Musk from Kamrup was considered the best, from Nepal of medium quality and from Kashmir inferior.

In India mostly term *Kasturi* is used for musk but in Sanskrit, other names like *mirgnabhi* (navel of deer), *mrigmad* (euphoric deer) are also used. In Persian, it is called *mushk* (fragrance), which changed into *misk* in Arabic and from there musk in English.

The musk deer inhabits in cold climate, and earlier the deer was common in the alpine zone of the Indian Himalayas, China and some parts of Russia, but is at the verge of extinction in most parts of the world. It has been domesticated in China, where musk is obtained by surgical procedures without harming the animals.

Musk deer is the smallest hoofed mammal, 7-18 kg in weight. It is generally dark brown in colour, mottled and speckled with light gray markings above and whitish markings on the ears, chin and thighs. It is shy, timid and usually remains solitary.

It differs from other deer in some respect. For example musk deer alone has gall bladders. It has no antlers but male have two tusk-like upper canine, 6-8 cm long. These point straight down. They are very narrow, pointed and have very sharp edge (Fig. 2). Females also have a sharp upper canine but they are smaller. In males, musk gland lies in shallow pouch on a disk between navel and sexual organ (preputial follicle) in the form of sac, four cm or so in diameter and 50-70 gm in weight. The front portion of this sac has an opening covered with hair, while the posterior part is shriveled and joins with covering of the penis. This pouch has several convoluted partitions, fatty in nature. Musk is formed during the rutting season, which is of about one month duration. At that time it is so strong in smell that it puts the animal itself in the euphoric stage and he moves around in the forest aimlessly and can be easily spotted by the hunter. In the pouch musk occurs in the form of grain. In the case young, old and sick animals, musk is of inferior quality, whereas in adult, healthy, mature male it is of very high quality. It is not formed till the age of one, in two years old animal it is about 6-7 gm and it is in the form of white resin. Generally after killing the animals, the musk- pouch is air dried in sun, wrapped in hair of the animal and sealed in leather pouches and stored in air- tight containers. The musk pod is mixed with extraneous materials to increase the weight.

There are three musk deer species: *Moschus moschiferous, M. chryogaster* and *M. sifanicus*. Out of these *M. moschiferous* is smallest deer. It is native to Siberia, northern Mongolia, Manchuria and Sakhalin. In most of the Indian literature, the Indian species has been identified as *M. moschiferous*, but in actuality it may be either of the two other species. *M. chryogaster* is found in the Himalayas, in central and southern China and in the north Vietnam. *M. sifanicus* occurs in the Himalayas, in central China, and in Myanmar (Burma).

In Indian trade three types of musk is recognized:

Russian: It is very feeble in smell

Assami: It is the best grade, granules are black in colour with strong, penetrating smell. It appears to be the *Kamrup kasturi* of Ayurvedic texts.

Chinese: It is most expensive because it is free from ammonia and the other unpleasant odours. It is collected in Tibet and exported to markets in China

Sometimes musk from Mongolia, north Manchuria and east Siberia is also available.

Musk is an oleo-resinous wax like substance, having cholesterol compounds, sex hormones, and many odorous principles, the main being muscone (muskone). The odour is penetrating and persistent. Musk is 10-20% soluble in alcohol and 50-75% soluble in water.

In India, genuine musk is very hard to get, if at all available it is mostly adulterated. The commonest method of manufacturing fake musk is by mixing one musk pod in large quantity of minced liver of animals, so that the fresh liver pieces absorb the fragrance of musk and on drying become granular. This mixture is then made into the shape of natural pods by using the translucent skin of the animals.

The role musk plays in human sexual system was known to ancient Indians so they considered it a supreme aphrodisiac to increase libido. In Ayurveda, it is also considered a strong stimulant, cardiotonic, nervous tonic, useful in meningitis, and respiratory problems. It helps in sudden collapse. It increases vascular flow. It was said to exhilarate the mind and stimulate brain, spinal cord, the peripheral nerves, leading to stimulation of urino-genital system. It is mainly used as nerve sedative in epilepsy, hysteria and convulsions in children, and as a cardiac stimulant in impotency. It induces sleep in insomnia caused by mental and physical fatigue. It is effective when applied on the skin and is said to rejuvenate all the systems of the body. As a cardiotonic a preparation *Chanderodya Vrihat Kasturi bharav* along with root of *Bala* is considered efficacious. Musk is also administered with honey, *Mrigmd asav* and *Makardhawaj*. For general depression pills made of 65 mg musk and 195 mg camphor are prescribed.

Musk is said to be hot in nature in Ayurveda so is not good for persons, who are of "hot type" and in the case of any side effect by its use such as headache cooling preparations like rose water and *banslochan* (bamboo manna) are used.

Some experiments (Nadkarni, 1954) have indicated that oral administration of 10-20 drops of musk tincture with 30 ml of water, to the patients of leukopenia, doubled leukocytes, but in other experiments no such result were observed. Chopra (1958) after detailed clinical and pharmacological study of musk did not find much beneficial effected in it and concluded that whatever effects are may be due to its strong smell as is the case with valerian and asafoetida.

Now, in India, in place of pure musk either synthetic compound or the seed of *Hibiscus abelmoschus* is used. Synthetic musk is crystalline, pale yellow in colour and has a very mild, persistent, musk like odour. It is formulated from mixture of musk xylene, musk ketone, musk ambrette, musk aldehyde, etc. These compounds are not safe. In a study Japanese scientist observed that musk xylene cause liver tumour in rats. It does not get biodegraded easily, the carcinogenic levels accumulate and become dangerously high. Musk ketone damage gene in the chromosome.

REFERNCES

Chopra, R. N. et al. (1958) *Indigenous Drugs of India*. U.N. Dhur & Sons, Calcutta.

Nadkarni, K.M. (1954) *Indian Materia Medica*. Vol. II Dhoopteshwar Prakashan, Bombay

A14 *Mutilla occidentalis* (*Indergopa*)

Some author identify this insect as *Dasymutilla occidentalis*. It is known as *birbavati or beer bahuti* in India. It is a bright scarlet coloured 15-20 mm long insect with body covered with dense velvety hair. White and black varieties are also available but not preferred. It appears just before monsoon in the gardens, and is collected, dried, grounded and used as a saffron- coloured powder.

In Ayurveda, it is considered a nervine tonic in all types of weaknesses and is ingredient of some aphrodisiac preparations, particularly for external use.

This insect is very popular in *Siddha* and *Unani Tibb* systems of medicine where it is considered spermatogenic and a nervine tonic. It is said to be a good *Kaya kalp* agent as it protects the body from all types of toxins and saves it from senescence.

A15 URINE (*Mutr)*

In Ayurveda, great importance is attached to the urine of herbivorous mammals, particularly that of cow, sheep, goat, buffalo, elephant, camel, horse, ass and even of man for various treatments. In Susruta Samhita, one chapter is devoted to urine therapy. Carak has also spoken high of it.

Urine is an excretion of the body rich in waste products, but it also contains traces of secondary metabolites like hormones, minerals etc. The following ingredients have been reported from it per day from a normal healthy person (Free, 1975):

Alanine 38 mg

Argenine 32 mg

Ascorbic acid 30 mg

Allantoin 12 mg

Amino acids (total) 2.12 mg

Biotin 35 mg

Calcium 23 mg

Creatinine 1.4 mg

Cystine 120 mg

Dopamine 0.40 mg

Epinephrine .01 mg

Folic acid 4 mg

Glutamic acid 308 mg

Glycine 455 mg

Inositol 14 mg

Iodine 0.25 mg

Iron 0.5 mg

Lysine 56 mg

Magnesium 100 mg

Manganese 0.5 mg

Methionine 10 mg

Nitrogen (total) 15 mg

Ornithine 10 mg

Pantothenic acid 3 mg

Phenylalanine 21 mg

Phosphorus 9 mg

Potassium 2.5 mg

Protein (total) 5 mg

Riboflavin 0.9 mg

Tryptophan 28 mg

Tyrosine 50 mg

Urea 24.5 mg

Vitamin B6 100 mg

Vitamin B12 0.03 mg

Zinc 1.4 mg

The two important modern medicine derived from urine are Pergonal- a fertility drug and urokinase- a blood clot dissolver for unblocking coronary arteries.

Urine is said to have an anabolic effect on the body and also helps in expansion of spirituality. The quality of urine depends upon the type of food eaten. A vegetarian diet rich in fruits and vegetable is likely to produce less toxic substances and more nutritive metabolites which body cannot utilize at that time and are excreted out. By this urine intake, these nutrients are recycled in the body. This is the basis of the self–urine therapy. This treatment is considered panacea (*sanjivani*) even for diseases like cancer. It is said to help in *tridosha* and detoxification of the body. Lord Shiva was said to follow this practice, which helped him in a long disease free life. In *Shivambu Kal vidhi* a detailed account of this practice is given.

Before starting auto-urine therapy the patient is prepared mentally for this treatment. He is advised that instead of negativity he should think about the positive effects of the therapy. The treatment should start after careful testing of the urine of the individual by a health provider to see that urine is not contaminated with the toxins in the body and is fit for human consumption. The treatment starts with voiding the urine in clay or copper pot. The common practice of urine collection for medical purposes i.e. discarding the first and last flow and only collecting the middle portion, should be followed. The urine should be consumed immediately. The fresh urine is odourless and clear, the smell develops when it is acted upon by bacteria, after storage.

No food or drink is allowed for one hour of urine intake. All the foods, which are considered hot in nature such as, spices, sour (acidic) items are avoided and the patient is given balanced vegetarian diet only. Autourine therapy along with yoga exercises is said to impart a unique spiritual power to the body, and an aura develops around it. The body becomes healthy, active, strong and resistant to diseases and allergy probably due to development of auto-immunity.

Sometimes a mixture of distillate of five products, obtained from cow called *Panchgavya,* consisting of milk, yogurt, urine and feces and *ghee* is prescribed. The tasteless distillate so obtained and cow's urine is said to be good anti-microbial and anti-allergic agent. These build immunity in the body and improvement in some patients with AIDS has also been seen with this treatment. For clearing the arterial blocking, eczema, diabetes, jaundice (hepatotoxicity) cow's urine with salt and honey is prescribed. Cow's urine with *neem* (*Azadirachta indica*, leaves) is used for cleaning infected skin areas.

REFERENCES

Coen van der Kroon (1998) *The Golden Fountain. The Complete Guide to Urine Therapy.* Amethyst Books, Amsterdam

Free, A.H. (1975) *Urinalysis in Clinical Laboratory Practice.*

A16 YOGURT (*Matha, Dehi*)

An important product obtained after fermentation of milk is yogurt (*dahi*). In most of the earlier English translations *dahi* has been called curd but this does not seem proper. Curd is milk coagulated in the stomach (milk coagulum) so the correct term for *dahi* is yogurt, which is curdled milk containing lactic acid

Yogurt is well reputed since ancient times, because of its beneficial effects, it is used in all the auspicious ceremonies of *Hindus*, like *havan, yagya,* marriage, and is distributed as a *prasada* in the temples. In Ayurvedic texts *Caraka Samhita*, *Susrut Samhita*, and *Ashtang Sangrah* yogurt is considered *tridosha nashak*, anabolic for strength (*bala-verya*), and a nectar (*amrita*). It is a blood purifier, and stabilizer (cooling) for nervous and cardio vascular systems. Yogurt should not be eaten during night and is contraindicated for the persons with *rakta-pitta*, *sheet prakariti* and those with paralytic attacks.

The assimilation of yogurt in the body is immediate, whereas in the case of milk, it has to get fermented in the stomach for digestion. In the case of milk bioavailability of the nutrient to the body is twenty percent, while in yogurt it is 80%. During the preparation of yogurt by fermentation, the lactic acid bacteria, brings about great changes in milk so much so that in the end product (yogurt) the content of calcium increase by eighteen times. Milk may cause an increase in cholesterol in the body but this is not the case with yogurt so it can be used by the persons with heart problems and/or with a high blood pressure. It neutralizes the alkalinity in the intestine. It is a good geriatric tonic and prolongs life. Recently an isolate from extract of yogurt has been found to be useful in high blood pressure.

Yogurt contains citric acid, lactic acid, and hydrochloric acid. Lactic acid is antimicrobial and as an acid, regulates gall bladder secretion, acts as a liver tonic and helps in the proper function of all the sense organs. Citric acid acts as a blood purifier and provides immunity to the body against various diseases

In the patients where milk is contraindicated, *matha* can be used but in high fevers *matha* prepared from fat free milk and mixed with hot water, should be prescribed, as this type of patient cannot digest fat and cold *matha* may cause shivering. In diarrhoea it helps all those patients, which do not get relief even with the best medicines

Matha is anti-*tridosha* and is used in different ways in different conditions. In *vata* it is mixed with dry ginger (*sonth*) powder and rock salt (*saindhav namaka*). If a little powdered cumin and a bit of asafetida (*hing*) is added to it, then its good effect increase by many folds and it gives relief in piles and gastro-enteritis. In *pitta* problems, add sugar to *matha* but in vitiation of *kapha* use dry ginger, black pepper, long pepper and natural alkaline salts obtained from soil (*yavakshar*). *Matha* with *yavakshar* and dried sugarcane juice is also effective in urinary diseases.

It is contraindicated in extreme weakness, unconsciousness, hypochondria etc.

Matha when stirred and diluted with water, is made into following forms:

i) ***Ghol* or *adhrirka***: When yogurt is stirred with a little water to form a thin paste like consistency. It is digestive, retains fluids in the body, gives relief in *vayu* vitiation but increases *kapha*. To counter act its bad effect spices like asafoetida, cumin, black salt (a salt obtained by fusing *triphala* with common salt at high temperature) are added to it before use. In this way it becomes a good nutrient and provides relief in gastric problems.

ii) ***Mathit***: For preparing yogurt a common practice is to boil milk, let it cool till warm and inoculate it with a small amount of yogurt, shaking the whole mixture, and let it remain at a cold place overnight. In the morning an upper layer as a crust (*malai*) appears on freshly prepared yogurt, which mainly contains butter. It is scraped from above and the remaining yogurt is used. It is cooling in effect and helps in the cases of gastro-enteritis, piles etc.

iii) ***Takra***: For its preparation one part of yogurt with four parts of water is stirred. It is a bit hot in its effect and helps in sexual power. It vitiates *vayu* and helps in *kapha*.

iv) ***Udshrit***: In it both water and yogurt are stirred in equal quantities. It is said to have an anabolic effect.

iv) ***Chacika***:

When whole milk yogurt is mixed with a large quantity of water and churned vigorously, the butter separates from it and floats on the top from where it is removed. The remaining fat free fluid, yogurt milk is called *chach* or *chacika* or *lassi*. Commonly salt is added to it as per taste. It is cooling, gets digested easily, refreshes in fatigue and thirst. With the addition of common edible salt it prevents dehydration of body and increases digestive power. It is said to have a cooling effect on the body in summer.

It is sour, tasty and aids digestion. By its regular use relief is obtained in diarrhoea, indigestion, syphilis, and in inflammation of any type. It is very effective in loss of appetite, gripping, and restlessness due to congestion in the chest. *Chach* obtained from cow's milk is considered the best particularly for indigestion, where it not only gives relief but provides required nutrients also.

For the proper care of the digestive system and health of the whole body consumption of yogurt milk is highly recommended. It was postulated that with the wrong type of foods, like the present junk foods, prepared from refined starch, sugar, salt and fats, diseases of the digestive system arise more frequently. A person who does not have proper digestion or proper evacuation is always worried about his/her health, which leads to mental tension and stress. Yogurt milk can help in these cases by helping in proper function of digestive system. The ancient sages appreciated yogurt preparations very much and declared that whosoever uses *chach* never falls ill. It acts like nectar (*amrita*) in the body. It provides proper environment to the digestive system for the proper utilization of all the nutrients of the food. It stimulates the secretion of glands in the liver and gall bladder and acts as a diuretic. With its antimicrobial effects, it destroys those bacteria, which cause putrid smell in the body waste.

MARINE ANIMALS

A17 AMBERGRIS (*Amber*)

Known as *amber* in Ayurveda. It is an excretion of sperm whale, found floating in the red sea and shores of Africa. It is opaque, dark brown to ash gray, amorphous substance with musk like odour.

It is valued aphrodisiac from antiquity and is an ingredient of many multi- mineral Ayurvedic preparations like *Jawahar Mohra.*

As a stimulant, it is prescribed in sexual and nervous debility.

Ambergris is still a very important ingredient of many high- class perfumes. Its effect may be due to compound ambrox which now has been synthesized. Ambrox, is a high boiling C16 tricyclic ether

A 18 COWRIE (*Kauri*)

It is the shell of a marine mollusc *Cyproe moneta*, and earlier was used as unit of monetary system, like coins, for commercial transactions. The cheap items were traded in cowries and the expensive ones in silver and gold.

Cowrie is quite hard, and is used after calicination. Out of the various types yellow shell with a nodule on the outer surface and a weight of about 15 gm is preferred for medicinal purposes. These shells are first purified by suspending them in boiling lime- juice. These are then taken out and heated to obtain a *bhasam*. The *bhasam* is hot in nature but helps in the weakness of the digestive system.

A 19 PEARL (*Mukta, Moti*)

It is an animal product but considered a mineral, gem in Ayurvedic literature, because of its apparent resemblance to precious stones. Pearl can be differentiated from the minerals on the basis of their reaction to light. Mineral stone reflect whole light, while pearl partly absorb it, and partly reflect it. Pearls are soft (hardness 2.5 to 4) as compared to precious stones, which have hardness of 8-10, and can be scratched by a knife blade or piece of glass but not by a fingernail. Pearls are relatively strong and cannot be crushed easily. If foot of a man stamp on them, the natural pearl will bear such blows. They have a characteristic iridescence.

Pearl is a translucent and lustrous concretion formed by pearl mussel, or pearly oyster, inhabiting shallow sea and sand bank (Fig.3). A pearl takes about four years to form. Colour of the pearl depends on the secretion so produced by the animal it may be green, pink, orange and even black. The black pearls are the costliest. Pearls may be round, pea shaped, oval or irregular in shape, commonly 1-5 mm. The bigger and round pearls are very expensive. All natural and most culture pearls have minor bumps, pits or uneven colour or irregularity in growth. A perfect pearl rarely occurs in nature.

The various commercial varieties of pearl are:

1. Blister pearl: These are not true pearl as they are

attached to the outside the shell and not produced within the body of the shell.

2. Cyst pearl are perfect, round formed within the body of the oyster. These can be further divided into the following types.

Baroque: These are irregular pearls.

Cultured: It was seen that a pearl is formed within oyster by the deposit of layers on any particle so Japanese artificially introduced the particles in the oyster and got good quality pearl (Note: As per Indian mythology a pearl is formed by falling of a rain drop in the open oyster). Those pearls produced naturally by artificial introduction of a foreign body into oyster are called "cultured" pearl.

Cultured pearl is of the following types:

A) Whole cultured

B) Simulated blister pearl

C) Rice: artificially obtained by making an incision.

A pearl is formed by oyster by first producing a layer of a substance called conchiolin on a particle followed by layers of white nacre. The layers of nacre and conchiolin are stratified and secreted by a process of biomineralization, the layers are 100 microns to 1 mm thick, on a nucleus which may be a sand particle or any other small organism like parasitic worm or small matter of organic tissue. When a transection of a genuine pearl is studied under a microscope, numerous layers of argonite crystals joined by a cartilaginous albuminous matter conchiolin are seen. The argonitic material is translucent generally colourless to white. The organic material is opaque or black. The two types of layers do not alternate in any regular pattern but depend on vagaries of deposition also climatic and habitat during the formation of a pearl. The thickness and arrangement of the nacre and conchioilin determine the iridescence of a pearl. The luster of a pearl is a product of both of its shape, structure and composition.

In India pearls are mentioned in ancient repository of knowledge such as *Atharva veda*, *Samhita* and *Kautilya's Arthshastra*. In Ajanta and Ellora, the caves of Budhist era in south India, pearls like beads are quite often depicted on the coloured pictures.

In Indian sub-continent, since ancient times, Tuticorin (Tamilnadu in India) Gulf of Mannar and west coast of Srilanka were common centers for trade of pearls. Pearls in this area were obtained from *Pinctada radiata*, *P. maxima* and *P. margaritifera*, but gulf pearls were considered superior to these.

Rice crispie pearls were obtained from *Cristaria plicata* in China. Earlier these were collected from gulf area and the equatorial region, but now these pearl are commonly cultured in Japan.

The pearls which are longitudinal, irregular, conical, with depression or convulsion, black or lusterless are considered of inferior quality

ARTIFICIAL PEARL

These are manufactured in many ways but in a common method, the glass beads are covered over or filled with a resinous matter, pearl essence, obtained from fish fins. These artificial pearls can be easily detected by the absence of iridescence. By scratching their body and by removing the outer coating, their glass like nature is confirmed. Artificial pearls are heavier and are not affected by high temperature.

Composition of Pearls

The chief constituent of pearl is, 82-86% calcium carbonate, aragonite ($CaCO_3$) (the shells of all molluscs is also of calcium carbonate), a small amount (10-14%) of horn like albuminoid, and conchiolin ($C_{32}H_{48}N_2O_{11}$), and water 2-4%. The thin organic membranes, composed of conchiolin are interspersed through the aragonitic matrix of the pearl. Conchiolin consists of polysaccharide and protein fibers.

There are two mineral forms of calcium carbonate, calcite and aragonite, chemically both are identical but differ in the spatial arrangement of their component molecules, resulting in different physical properties such as hardness. Aragonite is more resistant to scratches and is heavier than calcite. Nearly all pearls are made up of aragonite. In addition to this the pearl contains the elements found in the water in which the oyster lived and may contain strontium and magnesium (both these elements are now considered good for human vascular system). Strontium occurs in higher concentration in pearls from sea-water than from fresh water.

The difference in strontium concentration and amount of organic matter in pearls can cause different reaction when the pearls are exposed to X rays and ultra- violet radiation. When natural fresh water pearls are exposed to X rays they usually fluoresce yellowish white where as natural marine pearls do not fluoresce at all. In contrast when natural marine pearls are exposed to long wave radiation, they usually fluoresce sky blue.

Like an onion, pearl contains concentric layers of organic matter. The presence of organic membrane in pearl makes it prune to both cracking and dehydrating. If the organic membrane dry out then outer layer of the pearl can peel off. The organic membranes inside the pearl are interlinked with aragonitic crystals. When subjected to high temperature calcium carbonate in the pearl breaks to calcium oxide- a chalky white substance. Pearls can also easily damage by acids or even acidic vapours. Therefore for preservation, enhancement of luster and surface protection, coating of the outer surface with beeswax, lacquer, buffering with chemical polishing compounds, coating with pearl essence made from fins of the fish, is commonly resorted to. These also fill cracks, pits, and holes etc

In ancient India genuineness of pearl was determined by the following tests.

1.Pearl is slimy to touch when rubbed with rice strand.

2. With salted cow's urine the luster of genuine pearl does not diminish.

Tooth test: It is quite common in the western world. In this the pearls are run gently along the edge of teeth. The genuine pearl because of organic nature will have a gritty feeling like sand dust at sea shore, while an imitation will have a smooth slippery feeling. Pearls can also be tested by their exposure to X rays. Imitation pearls are opaque to X rays and these appear white on the negative and black on positive photographs. The natural pearls are translucent, on the other hand, and appear gray on both negative and positive.

IN ASTROLOGY

Astrologically pearl is connected with moon. It increases emotional stability, mental strength, friendliness and contentment. It helps in weaknesses shown by anxiety, mental and emotional swings, worry, isolation, or the inability to cope with relationship with other people. For this purpose adoring the body with the biggest, natural round and beautiful pearl is said to help.

IN AYURVEDIC MEDICINES

For Ayurvedic medicine, small, deformed pearl which cannot be used for ornamental purpose are first purified by boiling with alcohol and lime water for three hours and dried in the sun for the whole day and whole night.

These are then used in the form of paste or ash, as in the case of coral, and the products so obtained is called *Mukta Pishti* and *Mukta Bhasma* respectively.

For making paste, pearl is macerated with cow's milk or rose water.

For ash (*Mukta bhasam*) a mixture of pearl and the other ingredients like mercurials, is incinerated in a crucible. Both preparations mainly consist of calcium carbonate and calcium oxide.

The best method of making a pearl paste is to take the discarded broken or deformed pearls of cheap variety, soak these pearls in lemon juice overnight till all the pearl dissolve in the juice. Wet the paste with clean water and remove all acid. Dry this paste. Beat an egg, mix the paste of the pearl in egg and use it.

Pearl products are good *Rasayana* (dose: 30-120 mg.) and are considered a good stimulant, tonic, aphrodisiac, nutritive, and sedative. It is commonly prescribed for the diseases of respiratory and sexual inadequacies. It is sometimes recommended to help in conception, and also to prevent abortion. It is a good source of bioavailable calcium to the body. It imparts longevity, is cooling to the body system, cools the internal heat, which cause inflammation of hand, feet, and other internal organs. It increases eyesight, vital energy, strength, and intelligence. It is astringent so checks bleeding and controls urination and helps in diarrhoea. It is a sedative, if used for 21 days, helps in irritation, apathy, thoughtfulness, hearing problems, mass phobia and other severe mental problems. It counter-acts the psychological imbalance caused by narcotics and hallucinogens. For wasting diseases use pearl preparations daily for two months with cow's milk. Earlier it was used along with mercurial preparations for tuberculosis.

Mukta pishti is an important ingredient of *Rasayana* preparations like *Jawahar Mohra*, *Kamdugdha Ras*, *Ramchura mani Ras*, *Suvaran Malini Vasant*, *Suvaran Vasant Malti*, *Vasant Kusmakar Ras*, *Vrahida Vangashwar Ras*, (For details of these see, Puri, (2003). In addition to these a preparation, *Mukta Panchamrit Rasayana*, used in wasting diseases and as a geriatric tonic, in chronic fever and tuberculosis, is prepared by taking 8 parts pearl ash, 4 parts coral ash, tin ash 2 parts, mollusc ash 2 parts, mother of pearl ash 1 part. Macerate these one after the other with *Pueraria, Asparagus*, aloe, milk, and fern *Adiantum* in a crucible. This product is considered a panacea if used for two months daily. Sometimes mercury and sulphur are macerated in lime- juice and added to the above recipe.

Another preparation is to take equal parts of pearl ash, coral ash, sulphur, and mercury. Mix sulphur and mercury in lime-juice and add rest of the ingredients. In chronic tuberculosis doze is 250 mg. It is said to provide nutrients to the respiratory system.

REFERENCE

Landman, Neil H. and Mikkelsen, Paula, M. Bieler, R. and Bronson, B (2001) *Pearl – a Natural History.* The American Museum of Natural History, New York

Matlins, A.L. (2002) *The Pearl Book: The Definitive Buying guide.* Gemstone Press, Woodstock, VT 05091

Nadkarni (1934) *Indian Materia Medica.* vol. II. Popular Prakashan, Bombay

Puri, H. S. (2003) *Rasayana – Ayurvedic Herbs for Longevity and Rejuvenation.* Taylor and Francis, London, New York.

A20 RED CORAL (*Monga, Parval*)

Red coral is obtained from *Corallium rubrum*, which is found at the base of deep Mediterranean-sea in big rock like coral reefs.

C. rubrum is a small gelatinous animal and the coral is obtained from its exoskeleton. The exoskeleton has main stump, branches and twigs. The thick part of this is used for jewelry but thin twigs, are preferred for medicinal purposes. Ancient Ayurvedic scholar considered it a mineral and not an animal, and it was included amongst nine precious gems.

In nature coral may be white, light brown, pink, red and black but as per Ayurveda, deep red, smooth, long cylindrical coral without any holes or branches is the best. After collection from the coral reef, the outer covering containing calcium layers and the other sediments are removed from the body of the animal and only red or pink part is collected, which after processing is deep red, waxy and smooth. It cannot be broken easily, fracture is horny and the whole body has same colour. It is non- combustible and can be differentiated from another product lac, which is also deep red in colour, is a resinous secretion of an insect and burns easily. Coral, which is dull in colour, light in weight, and is not rough, is not considered suitable for Ayurvedic preparations.

IN ASTROLOGY

In astrology coral is considered a stone for mars. It helps stimulate courage, energy, insight and ability to win over opponents.

IN AYURVEDIC MEDICINES

Before incorporating in any recipe. Coral is first treated variously. These treatments are called purification. In one of the processes, coral is boiled in the juice of *Amaranthus spinosus or Clerodendrum inerme.* If excess of calcium is sticking to it then it is cleaned with alkaline vegetables in special equipment called *Dola yantra.*

Pishti (Paste)

It is prepared by triturating purified coral twenty one times on wet stone with rose water. Paste is also made, by first boiling coral in milk, incinerating it, and then steaming it with rose water 21 times. The coral triturated in moonlight during the night, is called *Chanderputi* and that in the sun as *Suryaputi.*

Bhasam (Calcination)

For calcination, coral is first pulverized and it is then macerated in the pulp of aloe or the juice of *Asparagus racemosus* root, till homogenous. The mass is divided into small cakes using milk as binder, and heated in the furnace. This treatment is repeated three times till ash is formed.

In another process coral is first boiled in *Triphala* or with lime- juice, and is then subjected to heat in a crucible.

Coral after calcinations is ash like, mainly consisting of calcium carbonate, with small amount of magnesium carbonate, silica and iron oxide. In addition, coral ash may have numerous minerals found in its habitat.

THERAPEUTIC ACTIVITY

Coral is considered cooling, nervine tonic, sweet, alkaline, antacid, laxative and diuretic. It pacifies three *doshas*, it is antimicrobial, anti-dote to poisons and commonly prescribed in the diseases of respiratory and urino-genital system. Its common use is as a dilutant for the fast acting medicine to slow down their effect particularly as in *pittaj vikars*. Because of its cooling effect it helps in diseases, which originate in the body due to heat. In healthy persons it increases vital energy.

Coral is very rich in calcium. Coral calcium has recently been recognized as a good source of calcium for the body. One hundred fifiy diseases are related to calcium deficiency. It is called "king of minerals" but for bio-availability, body must convert calcium into organic form. When compared to other sources of calcium, coral calcium is superior with regards to absorption and bone density.

Coral calcium is absorbed by the body easily and thus helps in maintaining strong bones and healthy teeth. It clears kidney, intestine and liver. It alleviates insomnia, heart beat regularity and helps neutralize iron and harmful acids, and breakdowns heavy metals. It protects body from free radicals, and controls digestive system. It increases muscular and joint mobility, combats arthritis conditions, regulates blood sugar level and blood pressure. It is of particular benefit where foetus is not getting the proper nutrition, and expectant mother suffers from malnutrition. It helps if the lactating mother is week. It regulates the flow of blood and may help in hemophilia. For psychosomatic diseases, coral is said to act against nervousness and gives strength to the body to fight it.

In a detailed study for longevity in the island of

Okinawa in Japan, it was observed that it might be due to the use of coral calcium by the local population in that area. This product is said to give body a perfect pH, while supplying the basic ingredients for rejuvenation. It defies arthritis, osteoporosis, fatigue, insomnia and lack of mobility. It helps in natural ability to fight off diseases, helps in the prevention of risk of degenerative diseases. Scientists have discovered that a low level of oxygen in the body can disrupt the body's ability to function normally and at the same time can cripple immune system severely leading body's vulnerability to disease and premature ageing. Coral calcium can increase oxygen supply in the body, thereby reducing body- waste, which continue to build up. It boosts immune system, induces incredible feeling of well- being and increases longevity.

AYURVEDIC PRODUCTS

It is an ingredient of important Ayurvedic preparations like: *Rattivalabh Pak, Mukta Panchamrita Rasayana, Nari Kalyan Pak, Navratna Ras, Navratnkalp Amrit,* and *Jawahar Mohra.* In these preparations both *Parval Bhasam* and *Parval Pishti* are used. *Parval Bhasam* is strong (hot) in effect. It increases luster and gives strength to the body. It is particularly prescribed in chest diseases like cough, tuberculosis and copious perspiration. In wasting diseases it is given with ash of stag horn and starch of *Tinospora cordifolia* (*Gaduchi satva*). In high fevers, malodour, anemia, intense breathing problem, excess of sputum, heavy perspiration, in the morning, it is prescribed with processed gold and G*aduchi satva*. Doze 125-250 mg

Parval Pishti on the other hand is cooling in effect so is used in high fevers, *pitta* fever and to slow the metabolic rate, as an antihistamine, in burning sensation of the body and burning of hand and soles of the feet where it is administered with *Gullukand* (rose petals in syrup). In burning micturition it is used with rice water. It is a good haemostatic and stops bleeding in all organs. In tuberculosis, and the other wasting diseases the paste shows better results. Dose 60 -240 mg

Anna Parvala

In the Siddha system of medicine this preparation is prescribed

Ingredients: Red coral, ferrous sulphate, *Hibiscus rosa sinensis* flower, *Lawsonia alba* leaves and *Cynodon dactylon* whole herb.

By the use of this preparation, plasma cholesterol, LDL and VLDL cholesterol, triglycerides, phospholipids and free fatty acids were significantly reduced in the patients. The withdrawal of the drug led to slow increase in these lipids. Some patients were able to reduce their daily doses of antihypertensive and vasodilater drugs during this therapy. No side effects were observed.

REFERENCES

Shanmugasundaram,E.R.S., Sundram, P., Srinivas, K., Shanmugusundaram, K.R., Shankaran, J.R. (1991) Double-blind cross-over study of modified Anna Pavala Sindhooram in patients with hyperlipidemia or ischaemic heart disease. *Journal of Ethnopharmacology.* **31:** 85-99.

Naryanaswami, V. (1975) *Introduction to the Siddha System of Medicine.* Director, Pandit SS Ananadam Research Institute of Siddha Medicine, Chennai (Madras) India

Shastri, Kashinath (1994) *Rastringani* (in Sanskrit with Hindi commentary). Moti Lal Banarsi Dass, Varanasi 5 (India).

MISCELLANEOUS

MI *SHILAJIT*

It is one of the oldest, well- known organo-mineral compound of unknown origin in Indian subcontinent. In India the use of *shilajit,* is known since antiquity. It is said that *shilajit* purified and mixed with other herbs can cure any chronic or obstinate type of diseases. In Central Asia, where it is called *Moomiya* or *Mumie* it is mentioned in the medical texts of 95O AD.

Shilajit is a dark brown or black resinous substance emanating the smell of cow's urine. In the earlier English translation of Ayurvedic works, it is referred to as bitumen or bituminous compound, as it has black resinous bitumen like texture and was even named as *Asphaltum punjabinum*- which means asphalt from Punjab (a state in northern India), as it was mainly traded in the city of Amritsar in Punjab from the raw materials obtained from Himalayas and the other high mountains of central Asia. Earlier European worker considered it as extract of plant fossils, which have been exposed to sun rays.

In Sanskrit *shilàjit* means extract exuded from the rocks. It is said that it is produced due to the effect of heat of sun- rays on the rocks. In Ayurveda, *shilajit* of many types such as gold, silver, copper and iron has been recognized but all these types defy identification. It appears that they were different types of compounds, which had *shilajit* like properties. Out of these, the present *shilajit* appears to be that of iron type, which after purification, as per the traditional tests, is light blackish brown, lustrous, having smell like that of cow's urine. It burns without smoke and settles down in the water.

In India, *shilajit* is collected from high, arid, steep rocks in the mountains between 1000-5000m in altitude in Arunachal Pradesh in east Himalayas to the Ladakh in the west Himalayas (Jammu and Kashmir). It is also collected from China, Afghanistan and Central Asian Republics of former Soviet Union and Norway. The *shilajit* from all these areas varies as its composition is influenced by plant species involved, the geological nature of the rocks, local temperature, humidity and altitude.

It is well known in all the countries of it origin as a tonic and adaptogen for the human body in the adverse conditions. It is said that in erstwhile Soviet Union (now Russia) cosmonauts were given a regular dose of this compound before their space journey.

The exudes of *shilajit* (crude material) is collected along with rocks, coarse sand and is brought to plains of north India for purification. The simple method of purification consists of boiling the rocks with water to separate water-soluble and water insoluble compound, the later is discarded as it mainly consists of stones etc. The water-soluble portion is dried by direct heat or by sun- rays. The upper layer of *shilajit*, dried by sun- rays is called "*Surya tapi*" and is considered the best. Some author consider that *Surya tapi* is the one which exudates from the rocks in pure form by the action of the sun- rays (Tiwari, 1973).

In an another method of purification, the raw materials is placed in a drum of water, stirred vigorously and is kept overnight. In the morning the supernatant fluid is collected and dried to obtain *shilajit*.

Sometimes, crude *shilajit* is boiled with *amalaki* (*Emblica officinalis*) fruit or a mixture of three fruits *triphala* (*E. officinalis, Terminalia belerica* and *T. chebula*) or by a mixture of ten roots (*dashmula*).

There is a belief, particularly in Ladakh (cold desert area of Jammu and Kashmir state in India) that *shilajit* is the feces of mountain rats or beavers. It appears that these rodents eat *shilajit* and the other vegetable matter from the crevices of the rocks and pass most of it undigested during their winter hibernation, from where in summer it is collected by the local people. To confirm this observation, from Ladakh three types of samples were collected and studied. These were:

1. Raw - coarse lumps from mountain rock
2. Purified raw materials from rocks
3. Purified raw materials from the feces of the rats.

Organoleptically, these three samples were similar but varied when studied in details for the various constituents.

SOURCE OF *SHILAJIT*

Lal and Joshi (1978) and some European authors in the last century, considered *shilajit* as impure sulphate of alumina or an encrustation of aluminous shale on the rock, but the later studies showed that it predominantly consisted of organic compounds, which lead to speculation about its vegetable origin. From physical appearance it appears to be oleo-resin but the other extensive studies, where *shilajit* could be collected during summer months, pointed out that it is probably the dried latex of dendroid *Euphorbia* spp, the soft stem of which due to excess of sap and strong sun rays bursts in summer and mixes with the soil below. Pande (1973) considered *Euphorbia royleana* Bois as the source plant. During recent times, when chemical constituents of *E. royleana* were studied in both summer and winter, it was seen that the exudates of *E. royleana* and *shilajit* has the same chemical constituents in summer, both had sterols, triterpenes, aromatic carboxylic acid, ellagic acid, benzocoumarins and amino acids. Most of the above phytoconstituents were absent in E. *royleana* in winter, which strongly indicated that these compounds are formed in the summer by the action of strong sun-rays and ultraviolet rays which are common at alpine Himalayas. *Shilajit* has been reported in dry and arid western Himalayas and not from wet and humid eastern Himalayas. In western Himalayas it is exudated in the summer months of May and June and dry months of September and October. It may be due also to winds of very high velocity in this area, which create a xerophytic conditions, and dehydration so developed causes the succulent stem of *E. royleana* to burst. By this action the pulp from the stem comes out and spreads on the ground, which in conditions conducive to drying turns into a black mass. (*E. royleana* grows in the plains of India also but no such exudation takes place here, probably due to lack of atmospheric conditions prevalent at the alpine Himalayas.)

Russian researchers on the other hand considered junipers as the starting material for *shilajit* in the mountains of the central Asia. According to these authors the decomposed juniper berries got biotransformed by decades of exposure to sun and then seeped down into the rocks. After another 40-50 years the thick black paste was exuded from rocks by geothermal pressure. Gatherers scrap the paste from the rocks, clean the impurities to get a pure product.

Shilajit is often equated with *moomiya* of Central Asia, but in the literature of medieval times, another product obtained from human brain was also called *moomiya*. This product was made by hanging a young boy upside down, in such a way that his skull was just above the boiling water in a big pot. The skull of the boy was clubbed with a blunt weapon so that all the contents of brain and the blood fall on the boiling water and coagulate immediately. This dark brown proteinaceous resinous mass from human blood and brain was also used as *moomiya.*

USES IN FOLKLORE AND AYUYRVEDA

Shilajit is now generally used as a dietary supplement like other herbs as such or as an ingredient of the various formulations. It is a constituent of Ayurvedic preparations like *Navratnakalp Amrit*, *Rativallabh Pak*, and many commercial products. Sometimes it is used as a *Rasayana*, (Puri, 2003) under the supervision of an Ayurvedic health provider. In this case body is first cleaned by *Panchkarma* before sunrise during winter months, and a dose of 250 to 1500 mg (the dose mentioned in the earlier texts is too high and may not be digestible) with honey or milk, followed by after 2-3 hours, a preparation of milk, rice and barley, is prescribed. Use of barley is essential but that of a bean *kulath (Dolichos biflorus*), which contains an enzyme urease, a well known diuretic, is totally forbidden. If *shilajit* is used with *kulath* then the nitrogenous compounds of *shilajit* degrade making it ineffective. All food items, hot in nature or which generate excessive heat in the body (increases metabolic rate) are to be avoided, as *shilajit* is considered to induce hotness in the body (Tewari, 1973).

The forbidden items include spices, pepper, sour things, excessive exercise and sexual intercourse.

In ancient texts, it is stressed that milk must be used during the administration of *shilajit*. Milk may be helping in the metabolism of *shilajit* in the following ways:

With the use of *shilajit*, there is an immediate depletion of body fat and cholesterol. Milk provides the required nutrients and saves the body from the sudden shock.

It appears that the various constituents in *shilajit* work better in a medium of milk.

Probably *shilajit* gets bound with proteins or fats of milk and forms a complex compound, which has no side effect. *Shilajit* in bound form is released to the body slowly, which has a better bioavailability for a longer duration.

The persons who cannot tolerate milk are prescribed cow's urine or dilute solution of vinegar as a medium of administration.

Shilajit has been recommended for use for 7-21 days and 49 days probably keeping in view the bio-availability of it to the human system

USE IN AYURVEDA

As an anabolic agent

It is said to support muscle strength and power and helps in healing of skin and soft tissues. For this, grated fresh coconut is roasted slightly, and the juice of coconut recovered during grating, if any, is mixed in it. This heated coconut is boiled vigorously in four times milk, till dry. Add to it raisin, sugar, honey as per taste and 1 gm *shilajit*. Use this milk preparation as per the digestion power for 40 days.

As a rejuvenator and immunomodulater

It is a reputed *Rasayana* and is said to impart immunity to the body and arrests process of ageing, if used in any form.

As an anti-stress agent

In central Asian countries, it is mainly used for cold and high altitude stress. In Ayurveda it is prescribed in many recipes for stress related diseases such as blood pressure, mental and physical fatigue. In one such product 5 gm each of chopped *anatmul* (*Hemidesmus indicus*), black *sariva* (*Ichnocarpus frutescence*) along with 10 gm liquorice, is boiled in two cups of water till it is reduced to half. This decoction is given with 250 mg of *shilajit* followed by a laxative.

For urino-genital system

In Ayurveda, it is well esteemed for the diseases of the urinogenital system. For urinary diseases, such as burning micturition, polyurea, diabetes, 250 mg *shilajit* with a teaspoon of honey and *triphala* (a mixture of three fruits) is prescribed.

For irritation in urethra

A mixture of equal quantities of long pepper, cardamom seed and *shilajit* is used.

In polyurea

Two pills (250 mg each) made from equal quantities of *shilajit*, cardamom, and bamboo manna with honey are given in the morning and evening with milk or with a decoction of *Pedalium murex*.

For diabetes

Shilajit 20 gm, *Ptercarpus santalinus* 40 gm, turmeric 20 gm, and fenugreek 40 gm are pulverised together. Half teaspoon of the powder so obtained is given twice daily with the juice of whole fruit of *Eugenia jambolana.*

As a sex tonic

It is said to increase libido and sexual power

For sexual inadequacies: Triturate by moistening *shilajit* 20 gm, organic compound of tin 20 gm, organic compound of iron 10 gm, mica compound 6 gm and make pills of 250 mg. Take one pill in the early hours of morning and one pill late in evening with sugar containing milk.

As a mental tonic

For fatigued brain: Take 250 mg *shilajit* with one teaspoon of butter.

For brain workers for increasing memory and physical endurance. Triturate *shilajit* 25 gm, processed iron 10 gm, saffron 2 gm, *amber* 2 gm, and make pills of 125 mg each. Take one pill two times a day.

In case of headache due to mental and physical fatigue caused by heat in the body.

a) Triturate *shilajit* and processed tin 20 gm each, processed iron 10 gm, processed mica 5 gm and make pills of 250 mg each. Take one pill twice daily.

(The above preparation is also prescribed for premature ejaculation and nocturnal emission, when due to weakness in the brain).

b) Make a fine powder of *shilajit* 5 gm, and 20 gm each of starch of *Tinospora*, and root of *Rubia cordifolia*

20 gm. Take half teaspoon of this mixture with *Emblica officinalis* candy (preserve).

In slackness of liver

If function of liver is hampered by fatty meals, excessive drinking, constipation or indigestion take *shilajit* and processed iron 250 mg each, mixed with half teaspoon of *triphala* and drink with cow's urine (half cup).

As a geriatric tonic

In old age it is used for the diseases ranging from ulcers, asthma, diabetes and rheumatism. It is used to attenuate the cerebral functional deficits, including amnesia in geriatric patients.

For quick healing of wounds and fractures

The tribal people of Afghanistan use it for the injuries inflicted during rock climbing in the rugged mountains, and in general accidents. In Ayurveda, pills made with equal quantities of *shilajit* and *guggal* (*Commiphora wightii*) are prescribed with milk. A plaster may also be prepared with both of these ingredient and applied (Puri, 2003)

AYURVEDIC PREPARATIONS

Shilajit Vati

Ingredients: *Shilajit* 50 gm, *Commiphora wightii* gum 28 gm, processed iron and tin 7 gm each, processed iron pyrites 14 gm.

Method: Processed metals are triturated for the whole day, and then gum and *shilajit* are added to them till the whole mass becomes homogenous. From it, pills of 250 mg each are made and dried.

Dose: 2 pills before breakfast and 2 pills after two hours of dinner, with sweet warm milk.

Use: A good nutrient, considered panacea for all urino-genital diseases.

Lauh Shilajit Vati

Ingredients: *Shilajit* 80 gm, processed iron 20 gm, processed mica 10 gm and processed tin 5 gm.

Method: Triturate minerals, when mixed homogenously add *shilajit* paste, make pills of 125 gm each.

Dose: 1-2 pills twice daily with milk. Add sugar to milk, except for diabetic patients.

Use: Well renowned for help in sexual deficiency, physical endurance, and stamina, for diabetes, anemia, and as a geriatric tonic.

Note: It may cause constipation because of iron, in that case a mild laxative may be used but the regular bowl habit must be maintained.

THERAPEUTIC INDICATIONS AND PHARMACOLOGICAL STUDIES

As a general tonic

In Russia serious research has been conducted on *mumie* since 1910. After several investigations, it was used as a performance enhancer within the armed forces, for cosmonauts, and for restoration programmes of international level athletics. It was found to be a good biostimulator, which elevated the immune system and neurohormonal regulation, controlled oxidation-reduction processes and had a positive influence on the mineral metabolism.

As a brain tonic

The effect of *shilajit* on memory, anxiety, and brain was investigated, for palliative notropic and anxiolytic activity. It was quite effective on rat brain monoamine. With subacute treatment for 5 days a decrease in 5 hydroxytryptamine, 5 hydroxy indole acetic acid concentration and an increase in the levels of dopamine, homovanillic acid and 3 hydroxy phenylacetic acid was observed (Jaiswal *et al*, 1992).

As an anabolic agent

It showed significant tonic and anabolic effect on both physical and mental processes in the case of sportsman. It was found to be highly beneficial to athletes who could withstand joint and connective tissue stress. It considerably facilitated the complete long-term overnight recovery as documented by morning biochemical and hormonal blood and urine tests. It also showed growth promoting and restorative role.

Anti-stress effects

The antistress and adjuvant effects were evaluated through a battery of tests. It augmented learning acquisition and memory retrieval in laboratory- animals due to anti-oxidant defense provided against several reactive oxygen compounds. It provided complete protection to methacrylate against hydroxyl radical induced polymerization and acted as a reversible nitric oxidecaptodative agent. It induced a dose related increase in superoxide dismutase, catalase and glutathione peroxidase activity in frontal cortex and striatum of rats, which confirmed its use as *Rasayana* against oxidative stress and geriatric complaints.

The samples of *shilaji*t obtained from India, Nepal, Pakistan and Russia were studied, for CNS and anti-stress activity. Samples from India and Nepal produced statistically significant effect in forced swimming induced immobility, restrained stress and aspirin induced gastric ulcer, and augmented the learning acquisition and memory retention in old rats (Ghoshal *et al.* 1991). The observed neurochemical effect by *shilajit* induced a decrease in rat brain 5HT turnover, associated with an increase in dopaminergic activity, helped to explain observed notropic and anxiolytic effect of it.

Anti-inflammatory activity

The aqueous extract of *shilajit* is biologically active. The degree of anti-inflammatory activity 50 mg/kg is similar to 25 n.g/kg of betamethasone. It was found to be anti-inflammatory, analgesic in rats, and reducer of ulcerogenicity (Acharya *et al.* 1988).

Anti-allergic activity

The compounds, fulvic acid, 4c-methoxy-6-carbomethoxybiphenyl and 3, 8 dihydroxy-dibenzo-a-pyrone isolated from *shilajit* have shown this activity.

Hormonal effect

Shilajit has hormonal effect on fish as it increased the reproductive potency, and induced spawning (Khosa *et al.* 1972). It showed a gradual enlargement of ovarian follicles, enhancement in maturity of ova bringing about vitellogenesis, with formation of considerable yolk (Khosa and Chandrasekhar 1978).

Antiulcer activity

It reduced acid secretion in stomach, a dose dependent decrease in ulcer index was evident (Acharya *et al.* 1988). In stress-induced gastric ulcer, *shilajit* from India and Nepal decreased the volume of gastric secretion and acid output, where as *shilajit* from Pakistan and Russia did not have this activity.

In hypercholesterolemia

It prevented diet-induced hypercholesterolemia in rats (Sankhala *et al.* 1992).

As an immunomodulater

It was seen to posses cell stabilizing action, against a number of challenges and prevented degranulation of sensitized mast cells (Ghosh *et al.* 1989).

Notropic and anxiolytic effects

Shilajit caused decrease in rat brain 5HT turnover, and an increase in the dopaminergic activity. Schliebs *et al.* (1997) observed that at a dose of 40 mg/kg of the body weight for seven days, *shilajit* induced an increase in cortical muscarinic acetylcholine receptor capacity. It partly explained the coginition enhancing and memory improving effects of *shilaji*t, which has the potentiality of use in Alzheimer's disease.

As an antidiabetic agent

A polyherbal product with *shilajit* was tried in alloxan induced diabetic rats. It resulted in significant reduction in blood sugar levels and a significant increase in liver glycogen. This effect may be due to glucose homeostasis brought about by an increased insulin secretion from repaired/regenerated pancreas tissues, which may be responsible for the prevention of hepatic glycogenolysis (Mitra *et al.* 1996).

MODE OF ADMINISTRATION

As per the Russian scientists, for sportsman in the initial stages a short-term cycle of use (10-12 days) is required for reaching the stimulative (restorative and anabolic) effect. The cycle may be repeated 3-4 times after a 15-20 days break. The effects of this treatment include the activation of anabolic processes on molecular levels in the different organs. For high intensity training it should be introduced during the training periods at a dose of 150 mg for 2-3 times daily. The first course should be half hour before training, second half hour after the workout and the third at the bed- time.

CHEMICAL STUDIES

On the basis of the earlier studies Chopra (1958) reported gum, resin, fatty acids, albuminoids and a large quantity of benzoic and hippuric acid from *shilajit*. The black colour was thought to be due to manganese. Presence of albuminoids and hippuric acid in it indicated that it originated from some animal. The recent chemical studies, on the other hand have shown that the various constituents of *shilajit* are like soil humus, produced by interaction of plant constituents from plant exudates and debris by rhizosphere micro-organisms. These constituents can be grouped into humic (80-85%), and rest non-humic. The non-humic part contains low molecular weight organic compound.

Alam *et al.* (1980) carried out studies on both the raw and purified *shilajit*. The raw material on analysis give 70% ash, 25.7% water soluble matter, 1.12% total nitrogen and 0.55% urea, while the purified *shilajit* yielded 14.78% ash, 82.90% water-soluble matter, 7.25% total nitrogen and 2.9% urea. These authors could not detect hippuric acid from the *shilajit* samples they investigated, but found glycine and benzoic acids. After their detailed study, they ruled out any possibility of link between *E. royleana* and origin of *shilajit*.

Other studies indicate that humification of resin bearing plant was responsible for formation of *shilajit* as it contains about 80% of humus components. It has got organic residues that have lost their original structure due to rapid decomposition of organic matter in the environment. Spectroscopic studies showed that it was structurally similar to ordinary soil. The two component of interest in *shilajit* were found to be fulvic acid and humic acid. Fulvic acid has the lowest weight component containing uronic acids, phenolic glycosides and amino acids, while humic acid is composed of high molecular weight compounds and contains a high proportion of phenolics. It has been seen that biphenyl metabolites of *shilajit* get partially transformed into benzocoumarins. The most common compound is dibenzo-a–pyrone. Physiological activity of *shilajit* has been found due to this compound, triterpenes and phenolic lipids. Fulvic acid may have a physiological role acting as a carrier molecule for more bioactive smaller compounds. One percent aqueous solution of Indian samples of *shilajit* had pH 6.2, whereas that from Russia had a pH of 8.2. Fulvic acid in the various samples varied from 15.4% to 21.4%. *Shilajit* commercial products are now being standardized for benzopyrones and fulvic acid (Phillips, 1997).

Dr Sarymsakov of the Kirgizt Academy of Sciences reported that *shilajit* contained over 30 micro-elements, 10 metal oxides, 6 amino acids and many other phytoconstituents

TOXICOLOGICAL STUDIES

Shilajit did not produce any mortality in rats up to 1 g/kg i.p, but some commercial samples which were not properly dried before packing were heavily contaminated with fungal organisms such as *Aspergillus niger*, *A. ochraceous* and *T. roseum*, which are capable of producing mycotoxins. Unprocessed *shilajit* contains significant amount of stable free radicals, which can cause irrepairable cell damage. The concentration of free radicals in humic material increases as the ph is raised, hence *shilajit* should not be given to the ulcer patients who have a greater risk of developing cancer (Phillips, 1997).

ADULTERATION

It is often adulterated with querus gall, cow's urine, gum, resin etc. Extracts of many herbs resemble with it. Powdered charcoal is a common dilutant in capsules filled with *shilajit*.

REFERENCES

Acharya, S.B., Frotan, M. H., Goel, R.K., Tripathi, S.K., Das, P.K. (1988) Pharmacological actions of Shilajit. *Indian Journal of Experimental Biology,* **26(10):** 775-777.

Alam, M., Rukmani, B., Usman Ali, S., Purushothaman,

K.K. (1980) Studies on authentic Shilajit samples. *Bulletin Ethnobotanical Research*, **4(1&2):** 54-61.

Chopra, R.N., Chopra, I.C., Handa, K.L., Kapur, L.D. (1958) *Indigenous Drugs of India*. U. N. Dhur & Sons, Calcutta.

Ghoshal, S., Lal, J., Singh, S.K., Goel, R.K., Jaiswal, A.K., Bhattachrya, S.K. (1991) The need for formulation of Shilajit by its isolated active constituents. *Phytotherapy Research*, **5(5):** 211-216.

Ghoshal, S., Reddy, J.P., Lal, V.K. (1976) Shilajit: chemical constituents. *Journal of Pharmaceutical Sciences*, **65(5):** 772-777.

Jaiswal, A.K., Bhattacharya, S.K. (1992) Effects of Shilajit on memory, anxiety and brain monamines in rats. *Indian Journal of Pharmacology,* **24(1):** 12-17.

Khosa, D., Chandrasekhar, K. (1978) Shilajit induced spawning in catfish *Heteropneustes fossilis* Bloch. *Journal of Research in Indian Medicine Yoga and Homoeopathy,* **13(4):** 119-120.

Lal, V.K., Joshi, P. (1978) Silajitu- a vegetable product. *Journal of Research in Indian Medicine, Yoga and Homeopathy,* **13(3):** 28-36.

Lal, V.K., Pandey, K.K., Kapoor, M.L. (1988) Literary support to vegetable origin of Shilajit. *Ancient Science of Life*, **7(3& 4):** 145-148

Mitra, S.K., Gopumadhavan, S., Muralidhar, T.S. (1996) Effect of D-400, an Ayurvedic herbal formulation on experimentally induced diabetes mellitus. *Phytotherapy Research,* **10:** 433-435.

Phillips, P. (1997) Unearthing the evidence. *Chemistry in Britain*, **3:** 32-38

Puri, H.S. (2003) *Rasayana: Ayurvedic Herbs for Longevity and Rejuvenation.* Taylor and Francis, London and New York.

Sankhala, A., Mathur, P.N., Sankhala, A.K., Deshora, P.K. (1992) Comparative efficiency of Shilajeet in preventing diet induced hypercholestrolemia in Wistar rats. *Indian Journal of Clinical Biochemistry*, **7(1):** 45-48

Schliebs, R., Liebmann, A., Bhattacharya, S.K., Kumar, A., Ghosal, S., Bigl, V. (1997) Systemic administration of defined extracts from Withania somnifera (Indian Ginseng) and Shilajit differentially effects cholinergic but not glutamatergic and GABAergic markers in rat brain. *Neurochemistry International*, **3O**: 181-190.

Tiwari, V.P., Tiwari, K.C., Joshi, P. (1973) An interpretation of Ayurvedic finding on Silajitu. *Journal of Research on Indian Medicine*, **8(3)**; 53-60.

M2 WATER (*Jal, Pani*)

According to Ayurveda, the cool water stored over-night in an earthen container, cow's milk, pure honey and pure *ghee*, all or any of these used by *Rasayana* methods every day in the morning, restores youthfulness. According to some scholars water should be used by people with *sheet prakriti* (cool nature), milk for *pitta prakriti*, honey by *kaph prakriii* and *ghee* by *vata prakriti*.

Scholars are also of the opinion that a best treatment for youthfulness is drinking water at sunrise. It acts as nectar. One should get up before sunrise in the morning and drink water kept in a clay pot over night, by mouth or by the nasal cavity. This water makes a man intelligent, with eye- sight like that of snake. The body becomes smooth without any wrinkles, and the hair turn black.

GLOSSARY OF TECHNICAL TERMS AND AYURVEDIC NAMES

Technical term	**Ayurvedic name**
Abrus precatorius	rati
Acacia bark	kikar chal
Acacia nilotica	kikar
Achyranthes aspera	apamarga
Adhatoda vasica	vasaka
Adiantum	hanspadi
Agama agilis	reg mahi
Agate	gomed
Alhagi camelorum	janwasa
Aloe	gheekunwar
Alum	fitkari
Amaranthus polygamous	cholai
Amaranthus spinosus	"
Ammonium chloride	naushadr
Anacyclus	akrakara
Argemone mexicana	satyanashi
Asparagus	shatawar
Asparagus racemosus	"
Asparagus sarmentosus	musli, safed

Aspergillus niger	fafundi (fungi)
Aspergillus ochraceous	"
Azadirachta indica	neem
Barleria prionitis	katsarya
Bauhinia purpurea	kobidar
Bauhinia variegata	kachnar
Bennincasa hispida	petha
Boerhaavia diffusa	punernava
Bombax malabaricum	semal
Borax	suhaga
Brassica juncea	rai
Butea	dhak (palash)
Butea frondosa	"
Butea monosperma	"
Calamus	vach
Calotropis	aak
Calotropis procera	"
Camphor	mushkafoor
Cannabis	bhang
Cannabis indica	"
Cardamom	choti illaichi
Cassia fistula	amaltas
Castor spp.	jund bedstar
Celastrus	malakangni
Centella asiatica	mandukparni
Chalk	chuna
Chlorophytum arundinaceum	musali, safed
Cinnamon	dalchini

Cinnamon leaves	tejpat
Citrus lemon	nimbu
Clerodendrum inerme	bharangi
Clove	laung
Commiphora wightii	guggal
Corallium rubrum	monga lal
Cristaria plicata	moti
Crotalaria juncea	sanpushpi
Curculigo orchiodes	musli kali
Cynodon dactylon	doob
Cyperus scariosus	nagarmotha
Cyproe moneta	kauri
Datura	dhatura
Desmodium gangeticum	shalparni
Dill	sowa
Dolichos biflorus	kulathi
Dysmutilla occidentalis	beerbahuti
Eclipta alba	bhringraj
Embelia ribes	babring
Emblica fruit	amla
Emblica officinalis	"
Eugenea jambolana	jamun
Euphorbia	dugadhi
Euphorbia royleana	thuha
Fenugreek	methi
Ferrous sulphate	heera kasis

Ficus benghalensis	bargad
Ficus religiosa	peepal
Gecko verticillata	sanda
Ginger	sonth
Hedychium spicatum	shathi
Hemedesmus indicus	anantmul
Hibiscus abelomoschus	lata kasturi
Hibiscus rosa-sinensis	japa phul
Ichnocarpus frutescence	sariva
Indigofera tinctoria	neel
Iguana	sanda
Lacerta agilis	reg mahi
Laccifera lacca	lakh
Lapis lazuli	rajvarta
Lawsonia alba	mehndi
Lime	chuna
Linseed	alsi
Liquorice	malathi
Lodicea seychellarum	darayi nariel
Long pepper	peepali
Mabuia carinata	reg mahi
Mace	javitri
Mesua ferrea	nag keshar
Mica	abhrak
Mimosa pudica	lajwanti

Momordica charantia	karela
Moschus chrysogaster	kasturi mrig
Moschus moschiferous	"
Moschus sifanicus	"
Mucuna	kawanch
Mucuna pruriens	"
Musk	kasturi
Mutilla occidentalis	beer bahuti
Nardostachys jatamansi	jatamansi
Nigella sativa	kalaunji
Nutmeg	jaiphal
Ocimum	tulsi
Ocimum sanctum	"
Opium	afim
Oroxylum indicum	sonapatha
Orpiment	hartal
Paederia foetida	gandhprasarni
Pandanus odoratissmus	kewra
Paspalum scorbiculatum	kodrav
Pedalium murex	gokshru bara
Phaseolus roxburghii	mash
Phaseolus trilobus	jangli moong
Phyllanthus emblica	amla
Picrorrhiza kurroa	kutaki
Pinctada margaritifera	moti jeev
Pinctada maxima	"
Pinctada radiata	"

Pistacea gall	kakrasinghi
Piper betle	supari
Piper cubeba	chob chini
Plumbago zeylanica	chitrak
Pomegranate	anar
Potassium carbonate	jawakhar
Pterocarpus sanatlinus	lal chandan
Ptychotis ajwain	ajwain
Pueraria	vidari kand
Pueraria tuberosa	"
Realgar	manshil
Ricinus communis	arand
Rubia cordifolia	manjith
Saffron	keshar
Sandal wood	chandan lakri
Salmalia	semal
Salmalia malabarica	"
Santalum album	chandan
Saltpeter	kalmi shora
Semecarpus anacardium	bhilwa
Serpentine	zaharmohra
Sida cordifolia	bala
Silver foil	chandi vark
Sodium carbonate	soda
Sodium chloride	namak
Solanum jacquinii	kateri
Solanum nigrum	makoh
Sticus officinalis	regmahi
Sulphur	gandhak

Tamarind	imli
Tamarindus indicus	"
Terminalia belerica	bahera
Terminalia chebula	harar
Tinospora	gaduchi
Tinospora cordifolia	"
Trapa bispinosa	singhara
Tribulus terrestris	gokshru
Turmeric	haldi
Vanda roxburghii	rasna
Vateria indica	sarjak
Vigna spp.	rajmaha
Viveria zibetha	jabad kasturi
Walnut	akhrot
Withania	asgandh
Withania somnifera	"
Zizyphus	ber
Zizyphus jojoba	"

INDEX

C

E

Q

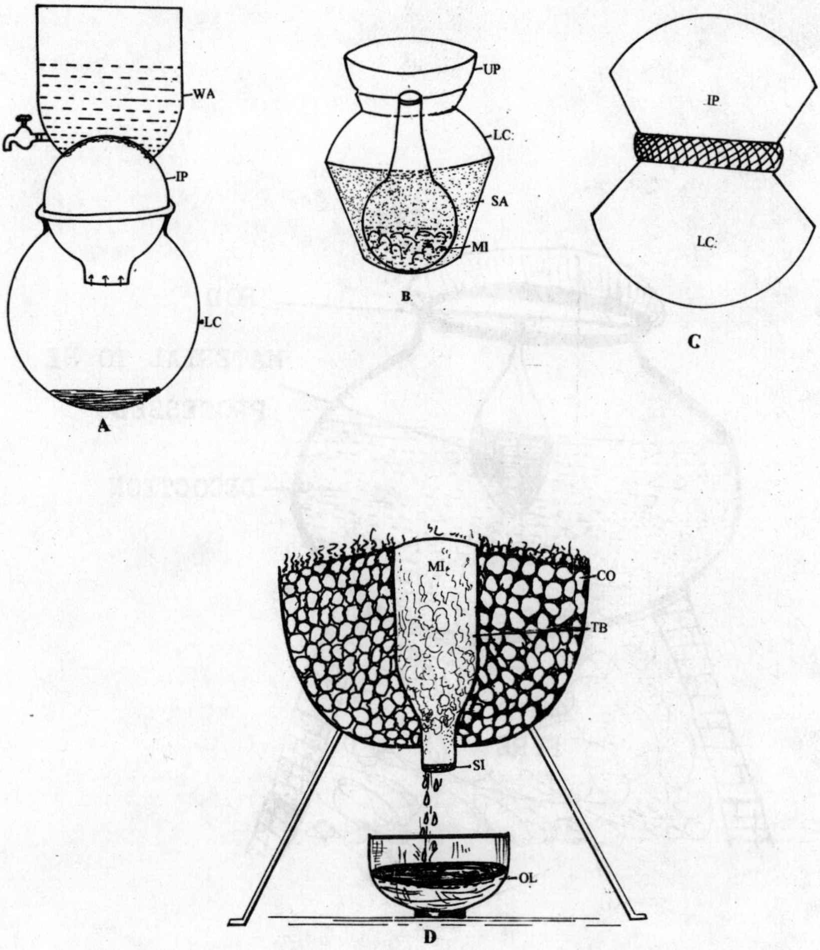

Figure 1 Equipment used for processing Ayurvedic products:
A. *Urdhavapatan Yantra*, **B.** *Baluka Yantra*, **C.** *Damru Yantra*, **D.** *Patala Yantra*.

Abbreviations: CO: coal, IP: inverted pot, LC: lower container, MI: material, OL: oil, SA: sand, SI: sieve, TB: thick glass bottle, UP: upper lid or container, WA: water.

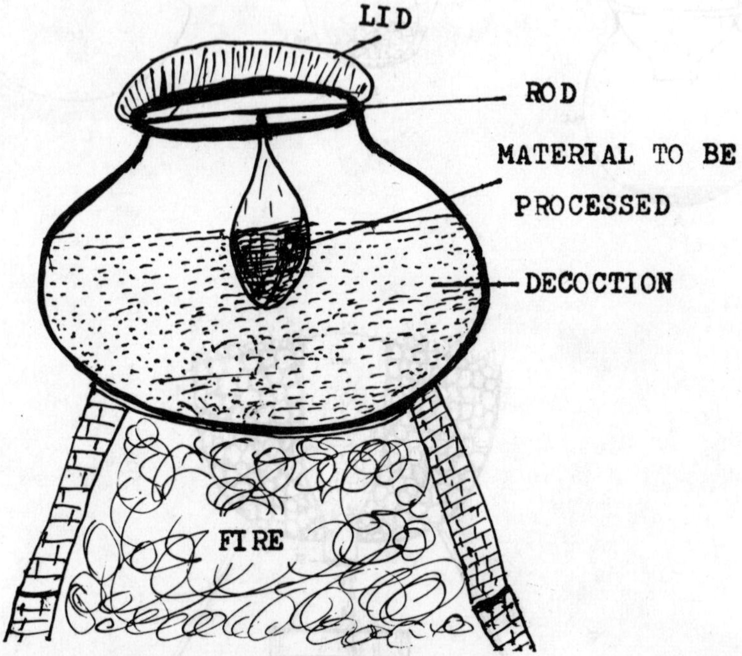

Fig. 2 *Dola Yantra*

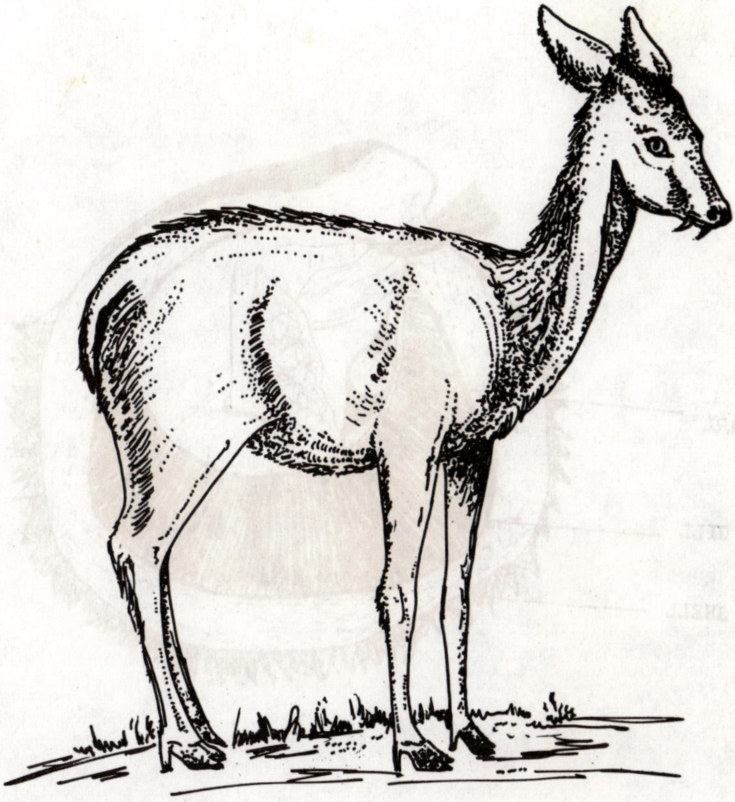

Fig. 3 Musk Deer

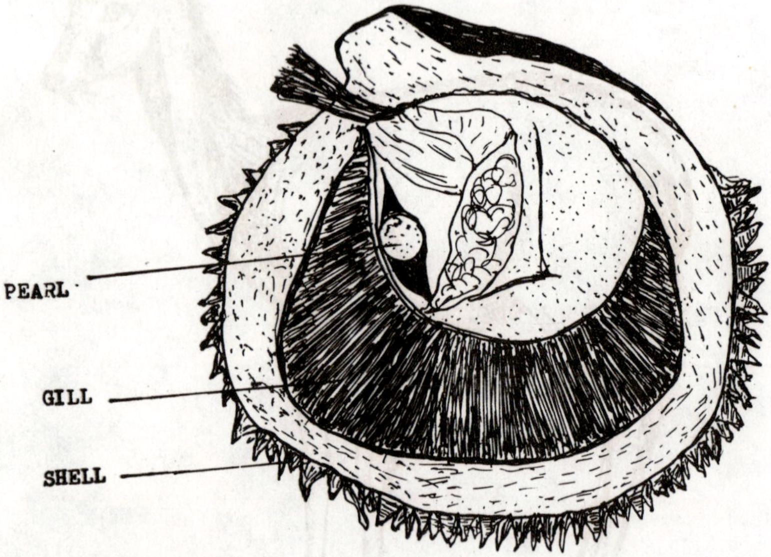

Fig. 4 Pearl oyster showing pearl.